Children's Health

Susan White

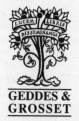

GEDDES &
GROSSET

The material contained in this book is set out in good faith for general guidance only. Whilst every effort has been made to ensure that the information in this book is accurate, relevant and up to date, this book is sold on the condition that neither the author nor the publisher can be found legally responsible for the consequences of any errors or omissions.

Diagnosis and treatment are skilled undertakings which must always be carried out by a doctor and not from the pages of a book.

Published 2008 by Geddes & Grosset,
David Dale House, New Lanark, ML11 9DJ, Scotland

© Geddes & Grosset 2008

Text by Susan White

ISBN 978 1 84205 614 1

Printed and bound in Poland

POLSKABOOK

Introduction

The aim of this book is to examine comprehensively topics that are relevant to children's health, from before birth, through adolescence to young adulthood. Subjects are described alphabetically and include some of the less common as well as the more prevalent diseases, illnesses and conditions of childhood. Aspects of mental health are described, along with other factors (exposure to sun, atmospheric pollution, smoking, alcohol, drugs, etc) which have implications for the health and wellbeing of children.

It is hoped that the contents of this book will be useful to all those who are involved with children. However, while the information contained is believed to be accurate, it is not exhaustive and a doctor should *always* be consulted if the health of a child is giving cause for concern. In many cases children, especially those who are very young, are more vulnerable than adults. People are occasionally reluctant to trouble their doctor over something that may turn out to be a trivial complaint. However, most doctors would almost certainly subscribe to the view that they would far rather see a child at an early stage, and so be made aware of his or her condition, than be called out some time later when the patient's health may have deteriorated. Hence if symptoms are a cause for worry, then this is a sufficient reason for calling the doctor so that the child may receive prompt and beneficial medical treatment. It is not appropriate to attempt to diagnose and treat a child at home unless it is obvious that the condition or illness is only a very mild one.

A

abdominal wall defects any of a group of disorders that arise during foetal development causing the baby's intestine to lie outside of the abdomen. During early foetal growth, the intestine develops within the umbilical cord but later it is normally enclosed by the abdominal wall. Rarely and for reasons that are unknown, this fails to occur and the intestines remain outside, appearing as a mass on the outside of the body. If the intestine has a surrounding covering of membrane, this is known as exomphalos. This condition is present in about 1 in every 3,500 newborn infants and it may be small or large. It is sometimes associated with other complications. If there is no surrounding membrane, then this even rarer condition is known as gastroschisis. Abdominal wall defects are emergency conditions requiring surgery soon after birth to make a repair. The extent of the surgery and length of the recovery time depend upon the severity of the defect, with all babies needing a period of special nursing and post-operative care in hospital.

abrasion *or* **graze** a superficial injury caused by the mechanical rubbing off of the surface of the skin (or of the outer layer of a mucous membrane). These injuries are very common in childhood. They occur from the moment a baby becomes a toddler and begins to explore his or her surroundings (with frequent falls) through to the time when he or she is rushing around on a bike or roller blades or engaged in energetic sports! Although most abrasions are generally not serious and can be safely treated at home, they can be painful and cause considerable distress. Hence reassurance is as important as treatment which consists of thoroughly cleansing the wound with warm water containing mild antiseptic solution, using clean cotton wool. The graze can then be gently patted dry, and some antiseptic cream and a clean dressing applied if necessary. If the wounded area is extensive, contains a lot of trapped grit or dirt or involves the face or head then it is necessary to seek medical advice. ANALGESIC (pain-relieving) drugs appropriate to the age of the child can be given if necessary.

acardia a very rare condition in which there is a CONGENITAL absence of the heart. It usually occurs in one of a pair of CONJOINED TWINS where one heart is responsible for the circulation of both infants.

acetone a chemical substance formed in the body when normal metabolism is upset, as during prolonged bouts of VOMITING, starvation, DIABETES MELLITUS and sometimes as a result of severe fever in children. The acetone is excreted in the urine (*acetonuria*) and in the breath, and in diabetes may be a forewarning of coma.

achondroplasia the most common form of DWARFISM, in which the long bones of the limbs are extremely short. This is because of an abnormality that results in permanent bone being formed prematurely so that normal growth is restricted. The bones of the skull are also affected, and the condition is inherited as a dominant characteristic that affects both the sexes.

acne neonatorum a skin condition that may arise in young babies, characterised by the appearance of spots on the face, generally on the forehead, cheeks and nose, and is caused by enlargement of the sebaceous glands.

acne vulgaris a common disorder of the skin, which is more prevalent during adolescence, especially among teenage boys. It is characterised by the eruption of pustules (pus-filled spots), whiteheads and blackheads which occur on the face, neck, chest and upper back and, if prolific, are unsightly and a cause of distress and embarrassment. The cause is an increased surge in hormones at PUBERTY, particularly androgens (male hormones), leading to over-activity of sebaceous glands in the skin which then produce greater quantities of sebum. Hair follicles become blocked and scratching leads to bacterial infection and the formation of the pus-filled spots. The surrounding skin is often inflamed, red and sore.

It is important to recognise that teenage acne, while not serious in a medical sense, can be an acute source of misery for a boy or girl. It occurs at a time when the young person is particularly self-conscious about his or her appearance and the unkind teasing of contemporaries is extremely hard to bear. Hence it must always be taken seriously and handled sensitively by parents. Over-the-counter preparations are highly successful in clearing up mild acne, along with careful attention to cleansing and drying of the skin and, above all, not squeezing the spots (to avoid scarring).

However, if the condition is severe the child should be treated by the family doctor who may prescribe topical preparations containing benzyl peroxide, tretinoin (retinoic acid), salicylic acid, vitamin A and/or clindamycin (an ANTIBIOTIC). Some cosmetic preparations aggravate the condition and need to be avoided. Also, it appears that certain (greasy) foods exacerbate acne in some people and it is best to reduce the amount of these in the diet. Sunlight can be helpful in clearing the condition and acne may be worse in the winter months in some cases. Rarely, in very severe cases, a skin specialist may prescribe a more potent form of vitamin A called isotretinoin (Ro-accutane), which is taken orally. However, in general, acne in adolescence clears up with time as hormone imbalances resolve and settle down as puberty progresses.

acquired immune deficiency syndrome (AIDS) a condition that was first recognised in the USA at the beginning of the 1980s. The causal agent was identified in 1983 and designated the HUMAN IMMUNODEFICIENCY VIRUS or HIV. The virus is found in blood and body fluids such as semen and vaginal secretions. It affects white blood cells, known as T-lymphocytes, which are vital to the effective operation of the immune system. Natural immunity declines, leaving the person increasingly vulnerable to the development of certain opportunistic infections and tumours associated with AIDS. In adults, it is transmitted mainly by sexual intercourse and the sharing of contaminated needles by intravenous drug users. Practising safe sex using a condom is one simple way of preventing infection among adults and a recent study has shown that male circumsion can reduce the risk of HIV infection in young men by up to 60 per cent. A number of years may elapse between becoming infected with HIV and the development of AIDS-related illnesses. The use of modern anti-retroviral drugs by people infected with HIV can further delayed the onset of AIDS for many years but controversially many of these drugs are not being made available to HIV-infected people in the developing world.

In children, the immune system is immature, and these illnesses may arise quite quickly and severely. Treatment is aimed at delaying the onset and controlling the severity of symptoms of any illnesses that may arise so that a child can lead as normal a life as is possible. Infants and children who are infected almost invariably became so during the process of birth. The virus is transmitted to the baby as it passes through the birth canal during labour and delivery. In addition, HIV has been detected in breast milk. However, modern drugs are highly effective at preventing HIV transmission during pregnancy, labour and delivery. When combined with other interventions, including formula feeding, a complete course of treatment can cut the risk of transmission to below 2 per cent. Even where resources are limited, a single dose of medicine given to mother and baby can cut the risk in half.

In the past (and still in the present in many communities), there has been an enormous stigma attached to HIV and AIDS because of fear and ignorance, and victims have been ostracised and made outcasts within their own communities. This is particularly sad when it has applied to children who have sometimes been excluded from playgroups, nurseries, etc, because of HIV. It is, of course, perfectly natural for parents to wish to protect their children from the risk of contracting a deadly disease. However, the HIV virus can be transmitted only by the direct mixing of infected blood or body fluid with that of a non-infected person. Ordinary family or social contact poses no risk. Children and adults unfortunate enough to be infected with HIV deserve the compassion and support of their circle of family and friends.

acrocyanosis *or* **peripheral acrocyanosis of the newborn** a bluish discoloration of the hands and feet of a newborn baby immediately after birth. It is a perfectly normal and short-lived condition.

acrodermatitis enteropathica a rare disorder that may affect babies, characterised by lesions and blisters on the skin and mucous membranes, failure to gain weight, DIARRHOEA and baldness.

acrodynia *or* **pink disease** (*also* **erythroedema**, **erythromelalgia**) a severe but rare disease of teething babies and small children in which there is pink coloration of the hands and feet, which feel clammy and cold. In addition, there is an itchy skin rash, copious sweating, red face, rapid pulse, sensitivity to light, digestive disturbances and loss of appetite. The child is at times extremely irritable and fails to sleep but this alternates with bouts of lethargy. The condition was more common when mercury was a constituent of infant teething medications and has become much rarer since this was banned. It has been suggested that the symptoms may have been an allergic reaction to mercury although this has not been scientifically proved.

acrodysostosis a rare, genetic disorder affecting the skeleton in which some bones fail to grow normally because they achieve maturity at an early stage. The bones most likely to be involved are those of the hands, feet and face, particularly the nose and jaw. The child typically has abnormally small feet and hands, an open mouth, a small nose and a jaw that appears too large. An affected child usually has accompanying learning difficulties. The responsible gene has not been identified but the condition appears to arise more commonly in children born to older fathers.

acromegaly *or* **gigantism** acromegaly describes a condition in which there is a great over-production of growth hormone from the pituitary gland, usually as a result of the presence of a non-cancerous tumour. The condition usually occurs in adults but if it arises in children who have not reached puberty, it results in rapid, excessive growth or gigantism. The condition does not only affect the skeleton but also soft tissues and organs. It may be treated by surgical removal of the tumour, radiotherapy and/or drugs to control the over-production of growth hormone. (*See also* DWARFISM, PITUITARY DWARFISM.)

acute childhood leukaemia *see* LEUKAEMIA.

acute epiglottitis *or* **supraglottitis** a severe inflammation and infection of the upper respiratory tract, which is of rapid onset and development and is most common in children aged between two and seven years. The condition can be fatal if the inflamed tissues swell and block the airway, and it is usually caused by haemophilus influenzae type-b bacteria or, more rarely, by streptococcal organisms. Symptoms, which generally arise quickly, include a sore throat, hoarse voice and high FEVER along with breathing difficulties. The child requires immediate medical treatment and is admitted to hospital so that a breathing (nasotracheal) tube can be inserted and the airway kept open. The child is also given appropriate antibiotics and supportive nursing care. Rarely, complications may arise and these include pneumonia or the involvement of the membranes (meninges) surrounding the brain and spinal cord or heart (pericardium).

acute infectious gastro-enteritis severe VOMITING and DIARRHOEA caused by a number of different bacteria, viruses or parasitic organisms. In some cases, the cause cannot be determined. Causal bacteria include *Staphylococcus aureus*, SALMONELLA and ESCHERICHIA COLI. Viruses that may be involved include some rotaviruses and enteric adenoviruses. *Entamoeba histolytica*, responsible for amoebic dysentery, is a common parasitic cause worldwide. Some infections provoke more severe symptoms than others, but infants and young children run a particular risk of developing DEHYDRATION and dangerous disruption of the fluid/salts balance within the body. Young children should always receive prompt medical attention as severe dehydration can arise within 24 hours. This may also be the case with an older child suffering recurrent bouts of diarrhoea and vomiting, especially if fluids are not being retained. A child showing signs of dehydration is normally admitted to hospital and may require fluids and electrolytes given by means of an intravenous drip. Appropriate ANTIBIOTICS may be given, depending on the nature of the organisms causing the infection.

acute infectious neonatal diarrhoea DIARRHOEA, often accompanied by VOMITING, in newborn babies caused by bacterial or viral infection. A baby may be infected by swallowing organisms present in the birth canal. However, in the home it may acquire an infection from the unwashed hands of family or friends, if strict standards of hygiene are not being adhered to. Outbreaks occasionally arise in hospital nurseries and nearly always occur by the faecal-oral route. Breast-fed babies are generally at lesser risk. As with all infants and young children, the main risk is that of DEHYDRATION. Unless the symptoms are very severe and the baby is too ill to suck, fluids and electrolytes are usually given orally. In serious cases, the baby may need to be treated in hospital with fluid and electrolyte replacement therapy. Breast- or bottle-feeding (with a specially prepared formula) is resumed as soon as the baby's condition improves to avoid the possibility of MALNUTRITION.

acute lymphoblastic leukaemia *see* LEUKAEMIA.

acute pyogenic arthritis a severe bacterial infection that may arise in one or several joints following a penetrating wound or injury. The condition usually arises in children and is accompanied by pain, FEVER, heat, swelling and sweating. Rest, antibiotics and supportive nursing care are needed until symptoms subside.

adactyly the CONGENITAL absence of one or more fingers or toes.

adenomeloblastoma a benign tumour of the upper jaw, occurring in the tissues beneath the teeth, which is most common in children or adolescents.

adenitis inflammation of one or more glands, which commonly occurs in childhood, particularly in association with upper respiratory tract infections.

adenoids a clump of lymphoid tissue situated at the back of the nose (in the nasopharynx). In childhood, they may become enlarged as a result of recurrent infections (*adenoid hypertrophy* or *adenoidal lymphoid hyperplasia*), and this frequently occurs in conjunction with swelling and inflammation of the tonsils (*see* TONSILLITIS).

In many instances, this is the cause of recurrent middle ear infections (OTITIS MEDIA), sinusitis, obstructed breathing, voice changes and hearing loss. These ongoing infections can, in severe cases, cause disruption to a child's schooling and a failure to thrive and usually necessitate surgical removal of the adenoids and tonsils in hospital. However, early treatment is normally by courses of antibiotics prescribed by the family doctor.

adolescence the period in the development of a child from the start of PUBERTY to the attainment of adult stature and the cessation of growth. It is marked by enormous physical, intellectual and emotional developments, which are usually more significant than those at any other stage in life.

adrenal gland *or* **suprarenal gland** each of the two kidneys within the body bears an adrenal gland on its upper surface. They are important endocrine organs producing hormones that regulate various body functions. Two of the most important of these are adrenaline and cortisone.

adrenal virilism an excessive secretion of androgens (male hormones) from the cortex of the adrenal glands which may be caused by the presence of a tumour or CONGENITAL ADRENAL HYPERPLASIA.

adrenoleukodystrophy (ALD) a rare, inherited disorder that is a recessive, sex-linked, metabolic and neurological condition affecting boys. It is marked by atrophy or shrinkage of the adrenal glands and degeneration of the brain and nervous tissue, resulting in a loss of speech and inability to carry out physical and intellectual functions. There is a defect in the action of peroxisomes (minute organelles within cells) that normally break down long-chain fatty acids by oxidation. It is the accumulation of fatty acids that causes the damage to the nervous system seen in ALD. The gene involved is carried on the X-chromosome and females can be unaffected carriers of the faulty gene. This is an extremely rare disorder and particularly tragic in that an affected boy develops normally during the first 4 years of life. But once symptoms arise, there is a steady and often rapid deterioration with very few sufferers surviving beyond the teenage years. A great deal can be done to help alleviate the symptoms and manifestations of early-stage ALD and, in the future, gene therapy may hold out some hope of treatment or cure.

adynamia episodica hereditaria an uncommon, inherited condition which may occur in babies that is characterised by periods of muscular weakness and floppiness.

agenesia corticalis a development disorder in an embryo in which certain brain cells fail to become differentiated. As a result, the baby is born with severe brain damage and mental impairment.

agenesis any failure in embryonic development which causes an infant to be born lacking the whole or a part of an organ.

AIDS *see* ACQUIRED IMMUNE DEFICIENCY SYNDROME.

air pollution in modern Britain this is a major factor affecting human health, and is a contributory cause of lung and respiratory diseases such as BRONCHITIS and ASTHMA. Children are very susceptible to these illnesses and recent studies appear to show that cases of asthma, in particular, are increasing at an alarming rate. The main elements of air pollution affecting children are vehicle exhaust fumes and cigarette smoking. Unfortunately, for those living in towns and cities, it is impossible to avoid vehicle exhaust fumes. The best that can be done is to avoid, whenever possible, venturing out with children at peak times of traffic build-up and to keep windows shut. Smoking is obviously a different matter and under one's personal control. Adults should be in no doubt as to the great harm they can cause to children if they choose to smoke (*see* SMOKING, effects on children).

akinetic seizure *or* **akinetic epilepsy** a type of seizure that may affect children. It is a brief episode in which the child becomes unconscious for a moment, loses muscle tone and collapses onto the ground.

Alateen an organisation that provides help and counselling for children and young people whose lives are affected by alcoholism in a parent or relative.

Albers-Schonberg disease *see* OSTEOPETROSES.

albinism a rare inherited disorder in which there is a lack of the pigment melanin in the skin, hair and eyes. A true albino has white hair, pink eyes and a pale skin and is very sensitive to light. The eyes are weak and vision is affected. A child born with this condition needs special care, in particular protection from the sun.

Albright's syndrome an uncommon metabolic disorder in which there is hormonal disruption that causes early PUBERTY in affected girls but not in boys. In addition, abnormal fibrous

13

tissue forms in bones and brown, flat spots appear on the skin.

alcohol – effects on family life, under-age drinking it is widely recognised that the child of a parent who has a problem with alcohol often suffers greatly before anything is done to relieve the situation. The child may be subjected to verbal, emotional and physical ABUSE, and have to carry out tasks or shoulder responsibilities well beyond his or her years. There may be frequent absences from school and consequent lack of achievement. In addition, the child is subjected to great anxiety and stress and misses out on many aspects of a normal childhood. All too often, the non-drinking parent and the family initially try to tackle the situation themselves and may be reluctant, from a sense of shame, to enlist outside help. This is particularly likely to be the case if the alcoholic person is repeatedly sorry and promises to reform but is unable to do so. Very often, a crisis point is eventually reached and the family is likely to need a great deal of help and support. Children benefit from skilled, professional counselling to help them to come to terms with the situation and the organisations Al-Anon and ALATEEN are of immense help in this respect.

During ADOLESCENCE, many young people are drawn to experiment with drinking alcohol and they may come under tremendous peer pressure to do so. Surveys have discovered that very many young people are drinking on a regular basis, at least once a week, and a significant proportion admit to having been drunk on at least one occasion. In spite of the fact that the legal age limit for the purchase of alcohol is 18 years, it seems that adolescents have little difficulty in gaining access to drink. Alcohol has a particularly potent and damaging effect in a growing person. It is absorbed rapidly and intoxication soon follows and, through inexperience, the young person fails to recognise when it is time to stop. Hospital accident and emergency departments are treating more and more young casualties of alcohol intoxication. Others have died due to inhalation of vomit while unconscious through the effects of drink, either abandoned or their plight unnoticed by equally intoxicated friends. Recent research has revealed that children who regularly drink alcohol are at far greater risk of becoming alcoholics in young adult life, compared to those who do not start to drink until they are older. Parents, teachers and adults in general have often felt helpless in trying to tackle the problem as, at this age, warnings tend to go unheeded. However, many believe that the best approach is to set an example of sensible and restrained enjoyment of drink in the home and that this is the place where a young person should be allowed to sample alcohol for the first time. Also, adults should educate youngsters about the unglamorous and ugly aspects of drinking to excess and all the misery that this can cause.

ALD *see* ADRENOLEUKODYSTROPHY.

ALL (acute lymphoblastic leukaemia) *see* LEUKAEMIA.

allergen any substance, usually some form of protein, that causes a hypersensitive, allergic reaction in a person who is exposed. There are a great variety of allergens which cause reactions in different tissues and body systems, such as the skin and respiratory organs. Examples include pollen, the droppings of house mites, dust and hair from domestic pets, some plants, drugs and foods.

allergic conjunctivitis an unusual irritation and reddening of the conjunctiva of the eyes caused by an allergic response and increased blood flow. Pollen, vegetation, various chemicals and cigarette smoke may be responsible and the condition usually occurs in children.

allergy a stage of hypersensitivity in an affected individual to a particular ALLERGEN, which produces a characteristic response whenever the person is exposed to the substance. In an unaffected person, antibodies present in the bloodstream destroy their particular allergens (antigens). However, in an affected individual, this reaction causes some cell damage and there is a release of substances such as bradykinin and histamine which causes the

15

allergic reaction. Many children suffer severely from allergies but, in some cases, these may subside with increasing age. The allergic response may produce respiratory symptoms – wheezing, breathing difficulties, blocked and runny nose, mouth ulcers, upset stomach – VOMITING and DIARRHOEA, or skin rashes, itchiness and ECZEMA.

Babies and small children may be allergic to a number of different kinds of food. Common ones include cows' milk, egg white, gluten contained in wheat flour and strawberries, along with many others. Food allergies are more likely to arise in a child of an allergic parent and also, twice the number of boys are affected than girls. A baby should be weaned very carefully onto solid foods which should be introduced slowly in extremely small quantities. If there is any sign of problems, the food should be stopped immediately. The child may be able to tolerate the food when he or she is older.

alpha fetoprotein a type of protein, formed in the liver and gut of a foetus, that is detectable in the amniotic fluid and maternal blood. It is normally present at low levels in the amniotic fluid. However, in a foetus with neural tube defects (SPINA BIFIDA and ANENCEPHALY), the level is elevated to an abnormally high degree during the first six months of pregnancy. This can be detected in a maternal blood sample around the 16th week of pregnancy and confirmed by AMNIOCENTESIS. If a foetus has DOWN'S SYNDROME, the level of alpha fetoprotein may be abnormally low. (Alpha fetoprotein is also produced by some adult tissues if the person is suffering from hepatoma, a type of liver cancer.)

alternating hemiplegia a rare and unusual condition in which a child experiences periods of muscular weakness down one side of the body. Following such an episode, the condition improves and the child recovers. During an attack, a typical feature is that there is variation in severity, frequently over a period of just a few hours and often there are associated problems such as difficulty in swallowing, eating, speaking and breathing. These problems may continue between attacks and about half of affected children also have EPILEPSY. Other movement disorders may be present and persistent, and learning difficulties are a common feature. The underlying cause is unknown but in many affected children, an attack is heralded by some warning signs such as excessive tiredness. In about 50 per cent of children, a trigger for an attack can be identified and factors include fever, emotional stress or excitement, high or low temperatures, bathing and common infections such as coughs and colds. Treatment is aimed at relief of symptoms and sometimes, hospital admission is required. In all cases, adequate sleep has been shown to be helpful along with avoidance of known triggers. Medication, including analgesics may also be prescribed.

alveolar bone grafts a surgical procedure used to repair a cleft palate and/or fistula (a hole between the mouth and nose). The part of the jaw in which the teeth are embedded is called the alveolus and it is abnormally split in a child with a cleft palate. In the absence of surgery, the teeth may either not erupt at all or arise in the wrong position. During the procedure a small amount of bone is removed, either from the child's hip or from the shin bone and this is grafted into place in the alveolus to bridge the gap. If a fistula is present, this is closed with stitches and finally, the gum is repaired to cover the bone graft and complete the operation.

amenorrhoea *and* **primary amenorrhoea** an absence of menstruation or monthly periods which is normal in girls before PUBERTY, during pregnancy and while breast-feeding and in older women after the menopause. Primary amenorrhoea describes the situation in which the periods do not begin at puberty. It is uncommon and may be caused by a failure or imbalance in the secretion of hormones. It also occurs in certain inherited chromosomal abnormalities such as TURNER'S SYNDROME or in the rare, congenital absence of the womb or ovaries. Many young girls who are developing normally become anxious if their periods seem late in starting, and worry that something may be wrong. It is important for girls to be reassured that there is a wide normal age range for the onset of menstruation (from about 9 or 10 to 16 or 17) and that problems are unusual.

amnesia, developmental a person suffering from developmental amnesia finds it difficult to remember single events that occur without any essential pattern or repetition and these include many events in everyday life. A child with this disorder may lose belongings or forget to take them and fail to pass on a message or run an errand, even when specifically asked to do so. The child may find it hard to follow a storyline in a book or film and is likely to become easily lost in unfamiliar surroundings. However, learning ability is generally unaffected as this is a memory disorder rather than an intellectual disability. The cause has been identified as being connected with damage to a particular area of the brain, the hippocampus, which is involved in long-term memory. It is believed that the hippocampus is particularly susceptible to oxygen deprivation such as may occur during a difficult birth or in very premature babies. Other causes may include fits and a disruption of normal heart rhythm. The damage to the hippocampus is permanent and irreversible but the child can be given practical strategies to follow to help overcome lapses in memory.

amniocentesis a procedure carried out to obtain a sample of the amniotic fluid surrounding a foetus so that it can be tested to detect the presence of such disorders as DOWN'S SYNDROME and SPINA BIFIDA. It is usually performed between the 16th and 20th week of pregnancy if there is a possibility of a foetal abnormality.

amnioscopy a procedure by which a small incision is made through the abdominal wall and womb of a pregnant woman so that an amnioscope (a form of endoscope) can be inserted to view the foetus. The procedure may also be carried out using a fetoscope inserted via the vagina and cervix.

amphetamines *see* DRUG ABUSE.

anaclitic depression a syndrome characterised by crying, refusal of meals, sleep disturbances and anxiety in a baby which has been separated from its mother.

anabolic steroids *see* DRUG ABUSE.

anaemia a condition in which the level of haemoglobin in the blood falls to an abnormally low level. Haemoglobin is the iron-containing pigment in red blood cells, responsible for transporting oxygen around the body. Haemoglobin levels can fall due to a lack of iron in the diet and this is the most common cause of anaemia in all children, with the exception of newborn infants. A further cause may be some defect or abnormality either directly affecting the red blood cells themselves or their production in the bone marrow. There are a number of diseases and conditions that can produce anaemia in children, including THALASSAEMIA or SICKLE CELL ANAEMIA, bone marrow disorders, CANCERS, especially LEUKAEMIA, certain inherited blood disorders, bowel and kidney disorders and haemorrhage. Symptoms include pallor, tiredness, PICA and shortness of breath. Diagnosis is made by means of a blood test. Treatment depends upon the underlying cause but may include dietary changes and iron supplements and possibly a blood transfusion.

anal fissure a break or ulceration of the tissues lining the anal canal which is quite common in babies. Symptoms include acute pain and bleeding with bowel movements. Surgery may be needed to effect repair if healing measures fail. The latter includes the use of suppositories to lubricate and protect the tissues and laxatives to soften faeces. These have to be used very cautiously in small children.

analgesic drugs many pain-relieving preparations designed especially for children have been developed over recent years and these are highly effective and widely available. Most contain paracetamol and are produced as pleasantly flavoured syrups which are acceptable to children. Children under the age of 12 years should not be given preparations containing aspirin because of a possible link with the rare disorder known as REYE'S SYNDROME. By the time they are 12, most children have mastered the knack of swallowing tablets and can safely be given a small adult dose of paracetamol at this age and above. It is very important to follow dosage guidelines, particularly with paracetamol which is highly dangerous or even fatal if taken to excess.

androgen one of a group of hormones which is responsible for the development of the secondary sexual characteristics and sex organs in the male. Androgens are steroid hormones and the best known example is testosterone. They are produced mainly by the testes but also by the cortex of the adrenal glands and, in minute amounts, by the ovaries of females.

androgen insensitivity syndrome (AIS) a rare, recessive genetic disorder carried on the X-chromosome which affects the gender of a child as there is abnormal development of the reproductive organs and genitalia. An affected child apparently has female genitalia on the outside but internally there is an absence of ovaries, fallopian tubes and womb, and testes are present. About one in every 24,500 children has this condition but it is not usually noticed at birth and it may only become apparent at puberty when there is a failure in normal female development. More usually, the presence of the male sex organs are noticed as INGUINAL HERNIAS and it is this factor that prompts diagnosis. Partial AIS describes a condition in which a baby is born with ambiguous external genitalia and may be designated either as a girl or a boy. In all cases, the psychological consequences can be profound and it is vital that both the child and parents receive expert guidance and help. As the child matures, surgery and/or hormone treatments can help to establish the gender identity in which the individual affected feels secure.

anencephaly a failure in the development of a foetus resulting in the absence of cerebral hemispheres of the brain and some skull bones. If the pregnancy goes to term the infant dies soon after birth, but spontaneous abortion occurs in about 50 per cent of cases. Anencephaly is often associated with SPINA BIFIDA and is the most common developmental defect of the central nervous system. It can be detected during the pregnancy by measuring the amount of ALPHA FETOPROTEIN present (*see also* AMNIOCENTESIS).

Angelman syndrome a rare, genetic disorder affecting about 1 in every 15,000 new born babies, caused by the absence of a gene on chromosome 15. The condition bears a number of similarities with PRADER-WILLI SYNDROME and causes severe learning difficulties and a characteristic appearance, notably a small head and particular facial features. Children usually have a sunny, happy personality and require educational and other specialist support throughout life.

anicteric hepatitis a type of very mild hepatitis that may affect babies and small children but usually resolves with time.

ankylosing spondylitis a progressive, inflammatory rheumatic disease affecting the spine and hip joints, characterised by stiffening and pain. It usually affects younger males, both adults and boys, and may begin as early as 10 years old. In the early stages there is lower back pain and stiffness, especially on rising in the morning. Later the disease progresses to involve the whole spine, and fibrous tissue replaces and fuses spinal discs and ligaments. Eventually, the whole spine may become rigid and the body bent forwards. There is no known cure but symptoms can be alleviated and exercise is important to maintain suppleness. However, care must be taken not to stress the back.

anorectal anomaly a developmental abnormality of the rectum and anus present at birth and affecting about 1 in every 3,000 newborn babies. It is more common in boys and there are two recognised types: low and high anorectal anomaly. With a low anorectal anomaly, the anus is either closed or it is abnormally narrow or displaced. With a high anorectal anomaly, the normal passage between the bowel and anus is closed but there may be a connection through to the vagina in girls or to the urethra in boys, through an opening called a fistula. In both types of anomaly, if there is a sealed passage present at birth then the infant is not able to pass meconium or faeces and so these build up causing abdominal swelling and vomiting. If a fistula is present, waste matter passes out through the abnormal route of the vagina or urethra.

Diagnosis is normally made soon after birth and an operation is performed to create an artificial opening (a loop stoma) so that waste matter can pass out of the body. At a later date and usually within the first 6 to 9 months of life, further surgery is carried out to close the stoma and to correct the abnormality. Depending upon the severity of the anomaly, a child may continue to experience some problems with the operation of the lower bowel following surgery. Hence periodic check-ups are required continuing into the teenage years, but most children can be expected to make a good recovery.

anorexia nervosa an eating disorder most commonly affecting girls and young women. It often begins in the teenage years but has been reported in even younger children. An anorexic child does not lose her appetite but has a false self-image and regards herself as fat which she finds abhorrent. As a result, she does not eat, exercise excessively, induces vomiting and misuses laxatives. Surprisingly, for some time the child remains active and able to carry on with normal life but loses more and more weight and presents an emaciated, skeletal appearance. This is accompanied by denial of feelings of hunger, secondary AMENORRHOEA, low blood pressure and hypothermia. The child may develop swollen ankles, vitamin and mineral deficiencies and extensive growth of downy body hair (lanugo) – the body's attempt to conserve heat. Usually there is severe depression and there may be attempts at suicide. If not cured, the anorexic person may eventually starve to death.

The cause of this distressing condition is unknown but anorexia rarely occurs in countries where food shortages and MALNUTRITION are commonplace. It appears to have a psychological basis but there may be other factors which make one person more vulnerable than another. Most young girls are aware of, and influenced by, the cultural idea of thinness which is perpetuated by the fashion industry. Many attempt to diet at some stage or another but very few become anorexic and it is believed that those who do have deeply rooted emotional anxieties and insecurities. These may relate to the family or, subconsciously, the child may wish to return to the pre-adolescent state and is afraid of attaining physical and sexual maturity. The anorexic may subconsciously feel that this is one means of regaining control of her life and receiving attention.

Treating anorexia is often difficult and is usually a prolonged process requiring considerable support and understanding from family and friends. It is often necessary for the young person to be admitted to a residential unit specialising in the treatment of eating disorders. Counselling and psychotherapy are an important part of treatment along with building up the person's weight. In order to save life, it is sometimes necessary for a person to be committed to hospital under the Mental Health Act and be force fed via a nasogastric tube. About half of anorexics eventually make a complete recovery while others improve but remain vulnerable. Between 10 and 15 per cent of sufferers die, some as a result of suicide. Unfortunately, the periods of prolonged starvation associated with anorexia can cause severe and lasting damage to body organs, particularly the heart.

antenatal before birth, referring to the health care given to a pregnant woman and her unborn baby.

antibiotic a drug that kills or inhibits the multiplication of disease-causing pathogens, usually bacteria. Antibiotics commonly given to children include ampicillin, amoxycillin, flucloxacillin and erythromycin. Doctors have to balance the benefits of giving antibiotics to individual children against the increasingly worrying problem of the development of resistance in pathogenic micro-organisms. An ill child will always be given the appropriate medication but parents should not expect antibiotics to be given routinely for very minor infections.

A child may have an allergic reaction to a particular antibiotic, which can manifest itself as a skin rash, fever, aches and pains or upset stomach. Fortunately, this is relatively rare and, if established, it is important that the child wears a bracelet or pendant that records the information. It should be borne in mind that antibiotics disrupt the balance of normal bacteria which inhabit the bowel and this, in itself, can cause symptoms such as DIARRHOEA but does not constitute an ALLERGY.

antibodies protein substances of the globulin type produced by the lymphoid tissue of the immune system and released into the blood. They react with their corresponding ANTIGENS and neutralise them, rendering them harmless. In a child, this reaction often produces swollen glands, e.g. in response to a bacterial infection. Antibodies are produced against a wide variety of ANTIGENS and these reactions are responsible for immunity and ALLERGY.

antigen any substance that causes production by the body's immune system of ANTIBODIES to neutralise their effect. Antigens are usually protein substances, regarded as foreign and invading by the body which provokes the antibody response. In the case of ALLERGIES, the antigens responsible are called ALLERGENS.

Apert syndrome an extremely rare, congenital, genetic disorder that causes the bones of the face and skull to fuse together (craniosynositosis) at an early stage in development causing distortion. Other common associated problems include brain damage and raised intracranial pressure, fusion of toes and fingers (syndactyly), abnormalities of the eyes and ears, cleft palate, breathing problems, acne, organ abnormalities and learning disabilities. The gene involved arises on chromosome 10 and the origin of the abnormality is usually a mutation in the father's sperm.

Apert syndrome is more likely to occur in babies born to older fathers (those aged over 50) but the incidence is still low at only 1 in every 65,000 infants. Treatment, which includes surgery to keep the sutures of the skull open to prevent premature closure and pressure build up within the brain, begins early in life. A great deal can be done to alleviate the severe effects of the condition but an affected child and his or her family will require ongoing, specialist support from a variety of different sources.

apgar score a method of assessing the health of a baby immediately after birth, carried out at one minute and five minutes following delivery. Breathing, muscle tone, response to stimuli, heartbeat rate and skin colour are assessed and each awarded a maximum score of two points. If a low score is recorded, it indicates the need for further close monitoring and possibly special care for the newborn infant.

apnoea of the newborn a temporary halt in breathing, usually preceded by disordered, rapid breathing, in a full-term, healthy, newborn baby. This condition is quite common and can be registered by an apnoea monitor which sounds an alarm if the baby ceases to breathe. It normally occurs while the baby is sleeping during the phase known as rapid eye movement (REM) sleep. It is naturally alarming but is normally transitory and does not cause harm. Apnoea is much more common, and usually more serious, in premature babies in whom breathing may have to be restarted. It can also be a sign of some underlying disorder in the baby. Such infants are monitored and cared for very meticulously in a premature baby unit. The baby is not sent home until there have been no phases of apnoea for at least one week, once he or she has gained some maturity. The parents receive careful instruction in the care of their child, which may include the use of monitoring equipment in the home and techniques of cardiopulmonary resuscitation (CPR).

appendicectomy *or* **appendectomy** the surgical removal of the vermiform appendix, the standard treatment for APPENDICITIS.

appendicitis inflammation of the vermiform appendix, which, in its acute form, is the most common abdominal emergency in the Western world. The appendix is a blind-ended tube, about 9–10 cm long, projecting from a pouch, called the caecum, which forms the first part of the large intestine. Blockage and infection of the appendix are the causes of appendicitis, which is most common in older children and young adults up to the age of 25. It is rare in young children under two years old. Symptoms include abdominal pain, which often begins in the region of the umbilicus but may move elsewhere. The pain is severe and is worse with coughing, deep breathing and movement. There may be nausea, VOMITING, DIARRHOEA, loss of appetite and FEVER. Eventually there is abdominal swelling and tenderness and acute pain.

Appendicitis is often suspected if a previously healthy young person complains of these symptoms. A doctor should always be consulted, and treatment involves admittance to hospital for appendicectomy. A rapid and complete recovery is the normal outcome. Danger arises only if the condition is left untreated, as the appendix may become the site of an abscess, or may become gangrenous and rupture, causing PERITONITIS. This is extremely rare in Western countries with good health care facilities.

arrested development the failure of one or several stages in the normal development and differentiation of the foetus resulting in various CONGENITAL defects.

arteritis umbilicalis a rare inflammation and infection of the umbilical artery in a newborn baby, caused by bacteria, generally the one responsible for TETANUS, *Clostridium tetanu.*

arthrogryposis multiplex congenita a CONGENITAL disease of one or more joints in a newborn baby. The disease affects the joint and its associated muscles and nerves and there is stiffness, presence of fibrous tissue and degenerative changes.

ASD *see* ATRIAL SEPTAL DEFECT.

asphyxia of the newborn *or* **asphyxia neonatorum** the condition in which a newborn baby fails to breathe normally and requires immediate resuscitation. There are many reasons why the condition may arise, and it may begin before or during labour and delivery or develop after birth. Although it is vital to initiate breathing by resuscitation techniques, it is also necessary to stabilise the various metabolic disturbances that result from asphyxia.

asthma in childhood asthma is a chronic, ALLERGIC condition that often begins in early childhood, afflicting more boys than girls, although apparently becoming more prevalent in both sexes. It is characterised by recurrent asthma attacks as a result of breathing difficulties caused by a narrowing of the airways (the bronchi and bronchioles) leading to the lungs. The main symptoms are breathlessness and a wheezing COUGH that may be worse at night. The extent to which the bronchi are narrowed varies considerably, and this governs the severity of an attack. In a severe attack, the breathing rate increases considerably and is rapid and shallow. The pulse rate likewise increases. If very serious, the child may be so breathless as to render speech impossible and there may be signs of cyanosis, i.e. a bluish colour of the skin and mucous membranes due to a lack of oxygen in the blood. Symptoms may be made worse by the fact that the child is likely to be extremely distressed and frightened and it is very important to provide reassurance. In these severe circumstances, or in any asthma attack that is not responding to the usual controlling medication, emergency medical care in hospital is needed. Prolonged and repeated attacks, with no break in between, are called *status asthmaticus*. This is also a serious emergency that can result in death due to exhaustion and respiratory failure.

The day-to-day treatment of childhood asthma is one of management to avoid the occurrence of an attack. This includes avoidance of the particular substance (allergen) or conditions that trigger the asthma if it is possible to do so. Drugs used in treatment are of two kinds. Bronchodilators are used to dilate the airways, along with anti-inflammatory drugs, and both are usually inhaled using a variety of different devices. There is now evidence that for some children, playing a wind instrument can help to alleviate the breathing problems associated with asthma, probably by improving the efficiency of the lungs.

The cause of asthma is swelling and inflammation of the walls of the airways, and contraction of the muscles, so that the openings are narrowed. This can be triggered by numerous different allergens including pollen, house mite debris, dust, hair and feathers from animals and birds and airborne pollutants, e.g. exhaust emissions and cigarette smoke. An asthmatic child often has other hypersensitive conditions such as ECZEMA or HAY FEVER and there is frequently a genetic link with prevalence within the family.

A recent breakthrough in research (announced in 2007) offers hope of new treatments for child asthmatics in future years. A gene, designated ORMD13, has been found to be present at much higher levels in the blood of asthmatic children compared to that of non-sufferers. This provides the strongest evidence to date of a genetic effect in this condition and research is ongoing to examine other genes which may be acting in similar ways in the causation of asthma. In some children, asthma is triggered by exercise (EXERCISE-INDUCED ASTHMA) and studies have shown that this is quite common and sometimes goes undetected. Emotional and psychological factors – anxiety and stress – may also initiate an attack and can exacerbate symptoms.

asyntaxia dorsalis a failure during development of an embryo so that the neural tube does not close, resulting in such conditions as SPINA BIFIDA.

ataxia with telangiectasia (A-T) *or* **Louis-Bar syndrome** a very rare, recessive, genetic disorder in which the abnormal genes are located on chromosome 11. It may also occur spontaneously as a new mutation in the affected genes and therefore does not always have an inheritance basis. There is a deficiency of the enzyme ATP protein kinase which is normally involved in the repair of DNA and in the metabolism of immunoglobulin. The disorder affects about 1 in every 300,000 newborn babies and symptoms usually arise before the age of 2 years. They include progressive cerebellar ataxia (loss of coordination and move-ment control), slurring of speech, blank expression, drooling and recurrent infections of the upper respiratory tract and sinuses. Between the ages of 3 to 10 years, there is the appearance of telangiectasia on the skin, especially on the ears and chest and conjunctiva of the eyes; these appear as knots of red skin lesions caused by the permanent, fixed dilation of minute blood vessels. There is a high risk of malignant disease and the child is hyper-sensitive to the effects of ionising radiation.

There is no cure for the disorder but prompt treatment of infections is essential and sometimes preventative antibiotics are required. Avoidance of x-rays, high doses of vitamins, physio-therapy, occupational therapy and speech therapy are other strat-egies that may be helpful.

Affected children usually become wheel-chair dependent by the time they are teenagers and they generally do not survive beyond the age of 25 years. Death is usually caused by CANCER and/or respiratory failure.

athetosis the type of involuntary writhing, involving the hands, face and tongue, which may occur in children with CEREBRAL PALSY.

atopic eczema *see* ECZEMA.

atrial septal defect (ASD) a CONGENITAL defect in which there is an abnormal opening in the septum (a partition) which usually keeps the two upper chambers of the heart, the atria (*sing.* atrium) separate from one another. The condition varies in severity depending on the size and location of the hole. It is usually detected in infancy, after about one year of age when blood flow has increased, although may be apparent earlier. The effect is to cause an abnormal left to right shunt of blood which, if severe, causes eventual enlargement of the right side of the heart. Surgical repair is the usual course of treatment which is generally carried out in early childhood. (*See also* VENTRICULAR SEPTAL DEFECT.)

attention deficit disorder (sometimes more popularly referred to as HYPERACTIVITY) a syndrome of childhood characterised by inability to concentrate, poor attention span, lack of coordination, behavioural problems, learning difficulties and a reduced need for sleep. Such a child may behave wildly (hyperactivity) and may be described as being out of control, even at an early age. The condition appears to be much more common in boys and is difficult and exhausting for parents, especially since it remains something of a mystery. In some children, hyperactivity appears to be linked with additives in food, such as colourings used in sweets and drinks or other factors in the diet. When given an additive-free diet, some children show a remarkable improvement although this is not the answer in all cases.

Controversial drug treatments appear to improve the situation in certain affected children, but the long-term effects of these may be unpredictable and doctors may be reluctant to prescribe them. In other cases, children can be helped by psychotherapy and special education. Unfortunately, problems tend to continue through adolescence and into adult life with poor academic attainment, lack of social skills, difficulties forming personal relationships and depression. This is particularly likely in children who do not receive appropriate treatment and family and parental support. Hence it is important for the whole family to be fully involved in the child's programme of treatment and great improvements can certainly be made.

autistic spectrum disorders *and* **Asperger syndrome** a group of emotional and behavioural disorders that cause problems with communication, learning and the acquisition of social skills. The cause is unknown but there is a genetic link in many cases and a tendency for autistic spectrum disorders to run in families, with boys being more likely to be affected than girls. Siblings of an affected child are at 75 times greater risk of developing the disorder themselves. Other factors affecting brain development both before and after birth are also believed to be important. However, worldwide studies have tended to disprove the belief that there is a link between the MMR vaccination and a rise in the incidence of autistic spectrum disorders among children.

The disorders vary from slight to severe and children with ASPERGER'S SYNDROME have a milder form and have a normal or high IQ (intelligence quotient). At least 580,000 people in the UK suffer from some form of autistic spectrum disorder and it is believed that many milder cases go undiagnosed. There is no specific diagnostic test but recent improvements in diagnostic techniques are thought to be partly responsible for some of the apparent increased incidence among children. Characteristics of the condition, which usually become apparent in infancy or early childhood include:

- difficulties with speech and non-verbal communication – avoidance of eye contact, inability to respond to gestures or facial expressions, emotional aloofness and detachment
- problems with normal social interaction – the child prefers to be alone and lacks the ability to take part in imaginative play.
- development of abnormal, obsessive, repetitive behaviours and rituals (*see* OBSESSIVE COMPULSIVE DISORDER)
- learning difficulties
- poor muscular coordination and lack of control of fine movements.

A significant proportion of children (some 15 to 30 per cent) are subject to fits, and medication to control seizures can be given in these circumstances. But for most autistic children, special education and learning support, cognitive behavioural therapy, language and speech therapy form the mainstay of treatment.

B

Babinski's reflex a normal reflex response in infants up to two years of age. When the sole of the foot is stroked, the big toe turns up and the toes fan out.

barbiturate a type of sedative drug (*see* DRUG ABUSE).

Batten's disease a very rare, recessive inherited disorder affecting nerve cells that leads to a progressive loss of intellectual and physical skills and an early death. The condition is caused by the absence of an enzyme which breaks down substances within nerve cells. In Batten's disease, it is the abnormal build-up of these substances that causes symptoms to arise. The disease affects about 1 in every 200,000 newborn babies but in order for it to occur, both parents must be carriers of the abnormal gene although they themselves are healthy. The disease exists in several forms that differ principally in the age at which they become apparent and in the rate of progression. In the late infantile form, also known as neuronal ceroid lipofuscinosis or NCL Type 2 or Jansky-Bielschowsky type, an affected baby starts to show signs of disease in the first year of life. There is a gradual loss of all functions and death usually occurs by the age of 12 years. In juvenile Batten's disease, also called juvenile neuronal ceroid lipofuscinosis or JNCL or Spielmeyer-Vogt-Sjorgren disease, the age of onset is usually between 5 and 9 years. The progressive deterioration that follows may be quite slow and erratic and death usually occurs between the late teens and early thirties. Epileptic fits are a feature of Batten's and can be treated with medication. Other symptoms and disabilities can be helped in various ways and although there is no cure, every effort is made to give sufferers the best achievable quality of life. Pre-natal testing can now be offered and the condition is the subject of ongoing medical research.

BCG vaccine *or* **Bacillus Calmette-Guérin vaccine** a vaccine that is given to provide protection against TUBERCULOSIS. All school children in the United Kingdom are given a pre-vaccination skin test (Mantoux test) and the BCG vaccine is then administered to those showing a negative result. The usual age for this vaccination is around 12 to 14 years.

Beckwith's syndrome *or* **Beckwith-Wiedemann Syndrome** a rare, inherited disorder of newborn babies in which there is a lack of glucose in the blood (hypoglycaemia), overproduction of insulin (hyperinsulin), enlargement of the tongue (macroglossia) and umbilical hernia along with other abnormalities.

bed-wetting *or* **nocturnal enuresis** a common occurrence in childhood in which there is an involuntary passage of urine during sleep. Most small children occasionally wet the bed but usually this ceases with increasing maturity. In some children the condition is more persistent and frequent, and they can be helped by various training techniques, such as the bell and pad method. In the latter case, an electronic sensor detects the flow of urine and sets off a loud buzzer or bell which wakens the child so that he or she can go to the toilet. This conditioning technique is normally very effective in helping the child to achieve control.

If any child wets the bed, it is extremely important for the parents not to become angry or critical as this induces anxiety, which makes matters worse. A young child who wakens up wet is often very upset and needs care and reassurance. It is best to change the wet things and return the child to bed as quickly as possible, without much comment.

benign juvenile melanoma a raised pink spot, most commonly arising on the cheek, which may occur in older children, especially between the ages of 9 and 13 years.

Berger's disease a disorder of the kidneys that is more common in males than females and frequently appears in childhood. Blood and protein appear in the urine and there is a build-up of immunoglobulin A (a protein important in the immune system).

biliary atresia *or* **neonatal hepatitis** a condition that may develop in the first weeks after birth in which there is damage to the bile ducts, resulting in an enlarged liver and jaundice. Surgery is needed in order to correct the condition and establish the flow of bile.

birthmark *or* **naevus** an agglomeration of dilated blood vessels creating a malformation of the skin which is present at birth. This may occur as a large, port-wine stain, often on the face, which may be treated by laser, or a strawberry mark which commonly fades in early life. Birthmarks are usually left alone unless they are prominent and a cause of distress.

birth injury a physical trauma during the birth process which may cause lasting damage.

bladder defect any of various types of CONGENITAL deformity that may affect the bladder, and these normally require surgical correction at an early stage in the child's life.

Bloom's syndrome a very rare, inherited, recessive, genetic disorder which affects 2 in every 100,000 newborn babies who are Ashkenazi Jews. The disease is extremely rare in people of other ethnicity. The defect involves a gene known as BLM which is normally involved in the repair of DNA – a function which helps to protect the individual against cancer. Children with Bloom's syndrome have no working BLM genes and as a result, show a high susceptibility to all forms of malignancy. Other features include retardation of growth, very low immunity, telangiectasia (red lesions composed of fixed, dilated small blood vessels) occurring on the face and caused by acute sun sensitivity.

Blount's disease *see* OSTEOCHONDROSES.

blue baby an infant born with CYANOSIS (a lack of oxygen in the blood) due to a CONGENITAL malformation of the heart. The result is that blue (deoxygenated) blood does not reach the lungs to pick up oxygen but instead is pumped around the body. Several congenital abnormalities of the heart cause cyanosis and they usually require corrective surgery.

bonding the creating of an emotional link between a newborn infant and its parents, particularly the mother. Bonding begins immediately after birth when the baby is placed in its mother's arms. Eye-to-eye contact, cuddling and gently talking to the baby are the normal vital components of the process and occur quite naturally in most cases. A failure in the process which may occur, for example, if the mother suffers severe post-natal depression, is a situation which requires professional help.

bow legs *or* **genu varum** a condition in which the legs curve outwards, producing a gap between the knees when standing.

Bow legs can be quite marked in toddlers and a cause of concern for parents. However, the condition normally resolves by the age of one and a half to two years and requires investigation only if it persists or becomes more pronounced. (*See* OSTEOCHONDROSES, KNOCK KNEES.)

BPD *see* BRONCHOPULMONARY DYSPLASIA.

brain tumour in children, a brain tumour is usually CONGENITAL and results from some abnormality during development of the embryo or FOETUS. The tumour may be benign but can still cause severe symptoms because of its location. These include severe headaches, fatigue, VOMITING and nausea, tiredness, inability to concentrate and vision disturbance. Treatment may be by means of surgery or radiotherapy.

breast milk jaundice a condition that may arise in a young baby during the first few weeks of breast-feeding. A substance in the mother's breast milk inhibits a metabolic reaction in the baby's body so that there is a build-up of bilirubin (the pigment in bile) in the blood and the development of jaundice.

breech presentation the situation in which, just prior to birth, the buttocks, feet or knees of a baby are the presenting part rather than the head. A breech position is likely to cause problems and a baby in this position is usually delivered by CAESARIAN SECTION to avoid the risks associated with a protracted and difficult birth.

brittle bone disease *or* **osteogenesis imperfecta** an inherited disorder of the connective tissue resulting in the formation of bones which are unusually fragile and brittle and which break very easily. If present at birth, the baby has multiple fractures, is usually deformed and this severe form is called osteogenesis imperfecta cognita. A generally less serious form may develop later when a baby reaches the toddler stage, and this is called osteogenesis imperfecta tarda. This form may improve as the child grows older. Other associated symptoms may occur including transparent teeth, unusually mobile joints and dwarfism. There is little treatment that is effective.

brittle diabetes a former name for TYPE I DIABETES.

Brodie's abscess an inflammation and infection of a limb bone, usually caused by staphylococcus bacteria, which is most common in children and which causes degenerative changes in the tissue.

bronchiolitis inflammation and infection of the lower respiratory system, i.e. the bronchioles (the very fine tubes that branch from the bronchi and end in the alveoli of the lungs). The illness is most common in young children and infants and frequently occurs in epidemics. It is usually caused by respiratory syncytial viruses (RSV) or the parainfluenza 3 virus but there are other pathogens which are more rarely involved. Symptoms include wheezing, breathing difficulties, severe COUGH, lethargy and sometimes FEVER. The child may become exhausted so that breathing becomes shallow and there may be signs of CYANOSIS and respiratory acidosis. Fluid and infected material leak from the inflamed tissues and may cause collapse of the alveoli. DEHYDRATION may develop if the child is VOMITING or cannot be persuaded to drink.

Most children can be treated at home and recover within a few days. More severe cases, those with underlying conditions or who are judged to be at greater risk should be treated in hospital. They may require administration of oxygen, intravenous fluids and treatment with the anti-viral agent, ribavirin given as an aerosol. Antibiotics are only given if there is reason to suspect the development of a secondary bacterial infection. If the cause is respiratory syncytial virus, there is a risk of the development of pneumonia and the child is usually treated in hospital.

bronchitis inflammation and often infection of the bronchi, the two 'pipes' or air passages that divide off from the windpipe and lead, via smaller tubes, to the lungs. Children may suffer from acute bronchitis as a result of an infection caused either by viruses or bacteria. Alternatively, the bronchitis symptoms may be an ALLERGIC response akin to ASTHMA. Bronchitis frequently starts with symptoms similar to those of the common cold but then a wheezing, painful coughing develops, with chest pain, FEVER and the production of a purulent (pus-containing) mucus. The latter is not usually evident in a younger child as it tends to be swallowed rather than coughed up. The treatment depends on the cause and nature of the symptoms. Bronchodilators, expectorants and antibiotics may be prescribed by the family doctor and the child usually recovers at home within about a week to 10 days. Bronchitis is more common in children who live in poor (damp) housing or whose parents smoke. It is more likely to affect boys than girls, and children who are overweight or who have a family background of allergic conditions may be more susceptible.

bronchopulmonary dysplasia (BPD) a chronic lung condition that may affect newborn babies who nave needed mechanical ventilation, especially those who are premature and of low birth weight. Recovery tends to be prolonged and an affected infant may need months of intensive care. Surviving children are often more susceptible to lung and respiratory tract infections, especially in their early years.

brown fat a special type of fat found in newborn babies which has enhanced insulating properties.

buccal fat pad an accumulation of fat in the cheeks, which is present in young babies and is often called a sucking pad.

buphthalmos *see* CONGENITAL GLAUCOMA.

burns and scalds damage to the skin and underlying tissues caused by extremes of dry heat in the case of burns and moist heat in the case of scalds. Burns may also be caused by electric currents and chemicals. It is well known that babies and young children are at risk from these injuries in the home and vigilance and special precautions must be taken by parents to protect them. Even a minor burn is extremely painful while more extensive or severe injuries are extremely serious and an all too common cause of death, often through shock or infection. With serious burns, treatment usually involves a prolonged stay in hospital and probably a series of skin grafting operations. Unless very minor, a doctor should always be consulted if a child receives a burn.

C

Caesarian section a surgical operation to deliver a baby by means of an incision through the abdomen and uterus of the mother. It is performed when there is a risk to the health of the baby or mother through vaginal delivery, both as a planned and as an emergency procedure. A Caesarian section is believed by many doctors to be beneficial for the infant in that it is spared the physical trauma of the birth process and is delivered without the squashed appearance of some normally delivered babies. Others hold the view that vaginal delivery prepares the baby's lungs for breathing outside the womb and that a Caesarian infant may be more likely to require assistance due to its sudden entry into the world. Julius Caesar is traditionally believed to have been the first baby born by this procedure, hence the origin of the name.

Caffey's disease *see* INFANTILE CORTICAL HYPEROSTOSIS.

calcareal epiphysitis inflammation of the epiphysis (the head) of the calcaneus or heel bone. It usually affects children who are physically energetic or engaged in sports, in whom cartilage is present and the epiphysis has not fused to the bone. It causes pain and inflammation and the foot should be rested as far as possible, until the symptoms subside.

Camurati-Engelmann disease a genetic bone and muscle disorder, usually affecting the legs, causing varying degrees of weakness, pain and wasting. Symptoms generally improve once growth is completed.

cancer a widely used term describing any form of malignant tumour. Characteristically, there is an uncontrolled and abnormal growth of cancer cells which invade surrounding tissues and destroy them. Cancer cells may spread throughout the body via the blood circulation or lymphatic system, a process known as metastasis, and set up secondary growths elsewhere. Many forms of cancer do not occur in children and adolescents. Those which may arise, e.g. LEUKAEMIA, are described under their individual headings.

cannabis *or* **marijuana, hashish, hemp** is a substance derived from the Indian hemp plant in the form of a thick resin, and is an illegal drug under current law. It is smoked, either alone or with tobacco, to produce its effects, which include feelings of euphoria, relaxation, a perceived slowing down of the passage of time and heightened awareness. It is one of the drugs which may be sampled and experimented with by older children, particularly those who smoke.

Recent studies have shown that even infrequent smoking of cannabis can greatly increase the risk of developing a psychotic illness such as *schizophrenia* in later life. The risk has been quantified as being 41 per cent higher in infrequent users of the drug, rising to between 50 to 200 per cent in regular users, compared to those who have never tried cannabis at all. The findings have worrying implications for the future mental health of young people, 20 per cent of whom admit to being regular users of the drug. It is believed that 14 per cent of psychotic disorders could be prevented if smoking of cannabis were to cease. (*See* DRUG ABUSE.)

caries *see* DENTAL DECAY.

catch-up growth a phase of rapid growth following a period when growth was inhibited due to debilitating illness or malnutrition.

It is common both in premature babies and in children who have recovered from a fairly severe or prolonged illness.

cat-cry syndrome an unusual CONGENITAL, chromosomal abnormality in which a baby is born with a small head, widely spaced 'crossed' eyes and ears that are low-set and abnormally shaped. The baby has a mewing cry and frequently suffers from physical, intellectual and heart defects requiring special treatment.

cerebral gigantism an unusual condition in which a baby is abnormally large and heavy at birth and continues to grow extremely rapidly for the first few years of life. There is no apparent hormonal abnormality and eventually the growth rate slows and resumes a more normal pattern, usually about the age of 5 years.

cerebral palsy an abnormal condition of the brain that usually occurs before or during birth and results in severe physical, and often intellectual, disabilities. It is usually detected soon after birth or in early infancy and is present for life. Cerebral palsy may arise as a developmental defect in the foetus due to genetic factors or can be caused by a viral infection during pregnancy. A lack of oxygen during a difficult birth or other trauma are further causes. After birth the condition can result from HAEMOLYTIC DISEASE OF THE NEWBORN or a brain infection, e.g. MENINGITIS. CONGENITAL cerebral palsy is commoner in boys and the overall incidence is 2 to 2.5 per 1,000 births. Less commonly, the condition can arise after birth due to severe infection or trauma and this type occurs equally in both sexes. Symptoms vary greatly in their severity and in the degree of disability they cause. A newborn baby may be floppy and have difficulty sucking but characteristically, the child exhibits spastic paralysis of the limbs. Also, there may be involuntary writhing movements (ATHETOSIS), and balance and posture are adversely affected. Often there is intellectual and speech impairment and sometimes EPILEPSY. Treatment depends on the severity of the symptoms and the degree to which the child is adversely affected. Generally, the outlook is quite favourable and many children are able to enjoy a reasonably good quality of life. Treatment may involve some surgery but in the main consists of physiotherapy, occupational and speech therapy and special education. It is now considered best to encourage a normal and active life to the limits imposed by the disability.

CF *see* CYSTIC FIBROSIS.

chicken pox *or* **varicella** a highly infectious disease of childhood, caused by the *Varicella zoster* virus, that is normally mild and of short duration. A childhood attack confers lifelong immunity, although the virus may remain within the system and become active at some later stage in adult life as shingles. Symptoms generally appear after an incubation period of two to three weeks when the child usually becomes slightly feverish and 'off-colour'. Within 24 hours, an itchy rash appears on the skin, beginning as small, red spots but developing to become fluid-filled blisters which vary in size. These may occur anywhere on the body including the scalp, inside the mouth and throat, in and around the eyes and on the genital area. New spots erupt over several days, and they are intensely itchy but eventually form scabs that fall off after about one week. Larger spots may leave slight pock marks on the skin after healing but these are not disfiguring.

The child should be kept at home until all the spots have healed and no new ones are appearing. Treatment consists of warm baths and the application of soothing preparations, such as calamine lotion and 'after sun' lotions, to relieve itching. It is not necessary to keep the child in bed but he or she should be persuaded, as much as possible, not to scratch the spots as this can cause secondary bacterial infection and increase the likelihood of scarring. There is no need to call the doctor unless the spots are very troublesome, and most children make a rapid recovery. But medical advice should be sought if the child already has an underlying disease or disorder, in which case anti-viral drugs may be given if appropriate, or if he or she seems very unwell. Similarly, if a sick child, e.g. a leukaemia patient, has been accidentally exposed to chicken pox, the child's doctor should be consulted. In such special circumstances the child may be given an injection of immune gamma globulin to prevent the development of chicken pox.

child abuse the physical, emotional or sexual abuse of a child. The abuse is all too often perpetrated by a parent, close family member or other person in a position of trust and may go on for years without being suspected or detected. Without appropriate care, the child may literally be damaged for life, with victims finding it difficult to develop a sense of self-worth or form relationships in adulthood. In recent years, people in Britain have had to come to terms painfully with the fact that child abuse is much more common than many would wish to believe, occurring throughout the social spectrum. Having faced up to this disbelief, many believe that one way of diminishing the problem is for all people in a community to develop a sense of responsibility towards children by being prepared to speak up if they fear that something is wrong. There is a great deal of professional help available to victims and their families, with the aim of protecting children and restoring proper relationships, whenever this is possible.

childhood nephrotic syndrome a rare disorder of the kidneys affecting between 2 and 7 children in every 100,000 and generally arising in those aged between 2 and 5 years. Boys are at a two-fold greater risk and there is a higher rate of incidence among Asian children and those of Arab ethnicity. Children whose family have a history of suffering from allergies are also at greater risk. The cause of the syndrome is usually unknown in the majority of cases but the presenting feature is an abnormal loss of protein from the blood into the urine (proteinuria). This causes fluid leakage and collection within tissues (oedema), often noticed in the lower legs and around the eyes. Diagnosis is by means of a urine test to detect the presence of protein.

Treatment usually comprises a course of a steroid drug (prednisolone) which stops protein loss and consequently brings about a reduction in oedema. Some children additionally require treatment with diuretics and/or infusions of protein. It is quite common for the condition to recur (relapse), hence routine home-testing of the child's urine for the presence of protein is normally required. The steroid medication can cause certain side effects and these must be reported and monitored. In a small number of cases the condition fails to respond and these then require more intensive treatments.

childhood-onset pervasive development disorder a disorder that is similar in many respects to AUTISM but develops at a later age, between 2 and 12 years. It is marked by odd behaviour, such as withdrawal and aloofness, inability to make friends, development of strange mannerisms and patterns of speech, and performance of rituals. Treatment is similar to that given to autistic children.

childhood peptic ulcer an ulcer in the mucosal lining of the digestive tract that may occur in infants and children as well as in adults. Over half of children with a duodenal ulcer have another family member with the condition so there would appear to be a familial tendency in some cases. A peptic ulcer is not a condition that is associated with childhood and in infants and very young children may only be diagnosed if it bursts and bleeds. Other symptoms include VOMITING and pain that may be worse after eating or during the night, although this is not always apparent. Diagnostic tests involving barium x-rays and fibre optic endoscopy must be carried out in hospital. Treatment for children is similar to that for adults, with dietary modifications and drugs (e.g. cimetidine and ranitidine) being given until the ulcer heals.

childhood polycystic kidney disease (CPD) a severe but rare disease of the kidneys and liver that may be present at birth or develop in childhood or adolescence. If it is present at birth, affected babies generally do not survive for very long because of severe under-development of the kidneys and lack of renal function. Older children and adolescents may show more symptoms of liver rather than kidney disorder. Medical intervention can improve symptoms and lengthen the life span but death eventually occurs through kidney or liver failure.

childhood schizophrenia *see* SCHIZOPHRENIA IN CHILDHOOD.

choanal atresia a rare congenital disorder in which the nasal passage on one or both sides of the nose is abnormally blocked by tissue or bone. It affects about 1 in every 10,000 babies with girls at slightly greater risk of the disorder. If both sides of the nose are blocked, diagnosis is usually made soon after birth as the baby experiences breathing difficulties. But if the blockage is on one side only, it may not become apparent immediately. Treatment is always by means of a surgical operation to make holes through the obstructing tissue and to insert very fine tubes (nasal stents), which are then removed in a second procedure about 3 months later. Most children make a good and full recovery.

choking interruption of breathing and violent coughing caused by an obstruction in the airway. In young children, the obstruction is usually a piece of food or a small object. Choking is a recognised danger during infancy when so many objects find their way into the mouth. If coughing fails to dislodge the object, there is a risk of suffocation and it is necessary to act quickly. The child should be held upside down and struck firmly in between the shoulder blades in time with the coughs. This should be sufficient to dislodge the obstruction upwards and outwards into the mouth.

chondrodysplasia punctata a type of DWARFISM in which there is stunted growth, a snub nose and thickened patches on the skin. It is a rare inherited condition that is sometimes fatal.

chondrodystrophia calcificans congenita a rare inherited condition in which there are abnormal patches in the epiphyses (the heads) of the long bones, which can result in bone defects, cataracts, shortened fingers, DWARFISM and intellectual impairment.

chondroectodermal dysplasia a rare inherited type of DWARFISM in which the limb bones are abnormally short and there may be polydactyly (extra fingers or toes). There are also likely to be various heart and circulatory abnormalities.

chondromalacia foetalis a rare, lethal CONGENITAL condition that causes stillbirth. Chondromalacia is an abnormality of cartilage, which, instead of being firm, is soft and malleable.

chronic bullous disease of childhood *or* **chronic bullous dermatosis** *or* **linear IgA dermatosis of childhood** a rare autoimmune disorder (one in which the body's immune system attacks its own tissues) affecting the skin in which groups of blisters erupt in rings on the face, around the mouth and in the groin. The blisters vary in number but tend to recur in phases on the same areas of skin, causing discomfort and itching. Diagnosis is made by means of skin and blood tests and the condition is not infectious. It generally occurs in children aged under 5 years and treatment is aimed at preventing the blisters from becoming infected, using drugs such as sulfapyridine. Some children are given steroid treatment in an effort to prevent blister formation. Usually, the condition is self-limiting and improves within about 2 years with the blisters leaving no permanent scars or marks upon the skin.

chronic mucocutaneous candidiasis a rare disorder that usually arises in young babies but can occur in later childhood or early adult life. It appears to be connected with an inherited abnormality involving the immune system and is characterised by respiratory and other viral infections, and skin lesions.

chronic recurrent multifocal osteomyelitis (CRMO) a painful, inflammatory condition of the bones without infection and characterised by active phases and periods of quiescence. The shin, thigh and collar bones are the ones most commonly affected and generally, during active phases, several bones are simultaneously involved. Various tests and scans are employed to arrive at a diagnosis and these reveal 'hot-spots' of inflammation in affected bones. The cause is not known but it is believed that the disease may be either an autoimmune condition (one in which the body's immune system mistakenly attacks its own tissues) or a defect within the immune system itself. CRMO is uncommon and affects significantly greater numbers of girls than boys and usually arises around the age of 10 years. Treatment is by means of medication, especially non-steroidal, anti-inflammatory drugs (NSAIDs) but steroids may also be needed in some cases. Physiotherapy may also be required along with rest. Many children eventually enter a period of remission, although relapses can occur, and there is generally a good response to treatment. In some cases, the growth of bones can be adversely affected and this then requires further specialist treatment.

circumcision surgical removal of the foreskin (prepuce) in boys and part or all of the external genitalia (clitoris, labia minora, labia majora) in girls. In females, and usually also in males, it is carried out for religious and cultural reasons. Female circumcision is physically and psychologically damaging and can never be justified on medical grounds in a young girl. In boys, circumcision may be needed to remove a foreskin that is too tight and is causing problems with urination (*see* PHIMOSIS, PARAPHIMOSIS).

cleft palate a CONGENITAL developmental defect in which a fissure is left in the midline of the palate as the two sides fail to fuse. It varies in its extent but can involve both the hard and soft palate, nasal passages and upper lip (harelip). Surgical repair is usually carried out at an early stage in the child's life.

clinocephaly an uncommon, CONGENITAL abnormality in which the upper portion of the skull sinks in slightly rather than being rounded, i.e. is concave and not convex.

clinodactyly an uncommon CONGENITAL defect in which one or more fingers or toes are abnormally bent.

clubfoot *or* **talipes** a CONGENITAL deformity in which one or both feet are twisted out of shape. It may result from squashing of the feet while the baby is in the womb and is corrected by the application of orthopaedic splints in early life. The great majority (about 95 per cent) of cases of clubfoot are of the type known as *talipes equinovarus*, in which the foot is turned both inwards and downwards. More rarely, *talipes valgus* may occur, in which the foot is turned outwards, or *talipes varus*, in which it is turned inwards.

clubhand an uncommon CONGENITAL deformity in which the hand is abnormally broad and stumpy and the fingers are short and poorly developed.

CMV *see* CONGENITAL AND PERINATAL CYTOMEGALOVIRUS INFECTION.

coarction of the aorta a CONGENITAL heart defect in which there is an abnormal narrowing of a part of the aorta (the major large artery of the body that arises from the left ventricle and from which all the other arteries are derived). The symptoms vary according to the degree of narrowing, from heart and circulatory collapse in severely affected infants to headaches, lowered femoral pulse, light-headedness, muscle cramps, nosebleeds and fatigue in older children. Treatment is by means of surgical repair, which in some cases may need to be carried out in the first weeks of life.

cocaine *see* DRUG ABUSE.

coeliac disease *or* **gluten enteropathy** a wasting disease beginning in infancy, when a baby starts to be weaned, and present for life. The disease affects babies of both sexes and is an allergic condition in which there is an intolerance to gluten, a protein that is found in wheat and rye flour. Symptoms begin when a child is introduced to foods containing gluten. They include loss of appetite, failure to thrive, lethargy, weight loss, pale stools, flatulence, DEFICIENCY symptoms and, possibly, anaemia. There is damage to the lining of the intestines, which are then unable to absorb fat. Hence there is an excess excretion of fat and the production of the symptoms described above. Treatment consists of strict adherence throughout life to a gluten-free diet. Most infants begin to thrive as soon as gluten is withdrawn and are usually given a high-protein, high-calorie diet with vitamin, mineral and iron supplements, if needed. In some cases, there may be a family history of coeliac disease or a possible link with other allergic conditions. There are several similar diseases, including the range of disorders called sprue.

cognitive psychology the study of the development of all intellectual processes and language in children.

colds *see* COUGHS AND COLDS.

cold sores in children cold sores are small blisters that appear around the mouth, caused by infection with the *Herpes simplex* virus. Evidence suggests that most people are exposed to this virus during childhood but many acquire immunity and do not develop sores. The initial infection may not be noticed but it can sometimes cause a high fever, acute inflammation inside the mouth and extensive mouth ulcers, accompanied by general malaise. Following recovery, the typical cold sore lesions may appear at a later date, often triggered by emotional stress, exposure to cold, heat or bright sunshine or following fevers and illnesses. Avoidance of any known triggers is important along with application of anti-viral cream when sores appear. Sometimes, a tingling sensation in the skin is noticed before a blister appears. In rare cases, especially in children with eczema or in those who are ill and with low immunity, more severe skin lesions can occur which need more intensive treatment. Children have to be taught the importance of not touching or picking sores so as to avoid spreading the infection.

colic in babies a common condition in young babies, between the ages of about 2 weeks to 4 months, affecting the digestive system and caused by wind. There are cramping, spasmodic pains that cause the baby to draw up its legs and cry loudly, often for several hours and especially in the evening. Infantile colic can be extremely distressing and worrying for parents, who may need reassurance that there is nothing seriously wrong. It is best coped with by general measures to try and comfort the baby and, while extremely tiring for all concerned, it fortunately usually subsides after the age of about three or four months. To try to prevent colic, the baby should be 'winded' during feeding and prevented from overfeeding or taking milk too quickly.

colostrum the first fluid produced by the breasts of a mother after childbirth. It is a fairly clear fluid containing antibodies, serum and white blood cells and is produced during the first two or three days prior to the production of milk.

colour blindness a general term for a number of conditions in which there is a failure to distinguish certain colours. It is more prevalent in males than in females and is usually inherited. The most common form is Daltonism, in which reds and greens are confused. This is a sex-linked disorder, the recessive gene responsible being carried on the X-chromosome and hence more likely to be present in males. The cause of colour blindness is thought to be the result of a failure in the operation of cone cells in the retina of the eyes.

communication – talking and listening to children it has now been established that it is vitally important for parents to talk to their baby, from birth onwards, in order to encourage BONDING and the development of intellectual and language skills. This is not always a spontaneous response for parents, who may feel a little inhibited at first. In a short space of time, their efforts begin to be rewarded as the baby starts to vocalise in his or her own way, with words appearing towards the end of the second year.

The pre-school years, up until the age of 5, are recognised to be one of the most important phases of intellectual development in the child's life. Adults who have the time and patience to talk to and explain things to a child, to read or play with him or her and answer endless questions, play a vital part in this process.

As the child grows older and increasingly independent, it becomes equally important for parents to learn to listen to their child and to encourage him or her to develop his or her own point of view. Problems inevitably arise, particularly in the teenage years, which can easily become a period when there is some breakdown in communication. If a good relationship, based on talking and listening to one another, has been built up over the previous years, problems and difficulties are much more likely to be resolved.

complementary feeding *or* **supplementary feeding** an additional bottle feed given to a hungry breast-fed baby. This may occasionally be helpful, especially in the early days of breast-feeding, before the supply/demand pattern is established. A complementary feed may also help to satisfy a baby who is hungry in the first two days after birth, when just receiving COLOSTRUM before the production of breast milk.

complex cyanotic congenital heart disease one or more rare CONGENITAL heart defects that cause disruption of the blood circulation and CYANOSIS (a lack of oxygen). They are treated, whenever possible, by various surgical techniques to restore a more normal pattern of circulation.

conceptional age the age of a FOETUS calculated from the time of conception.

congenital the term used to describe diseases, conditions, abnormalities or anomalies that are present at birth.

congenital adrenal hyperplasia a group of enzyme deficiencies that result in a low level of cortisol production from the adrenal glands. The pituitary gland at the base of the brain responds by increasing its secretion of adrenocorticotrophic hormone (ACTH), which has a stimulating effect on the adrenal glands, causing them to enlarge. The adrenal glands secrete increased quantities of the precursors of cortisol and of androgens (male hormones). During development, this causes masculinisation of the external genitalia of a female foetus (pseudohermaphroditism) and enlargement of the penis in a male. After birth, the imbalance causes a child to grow at a rapid rate at first but maturation of the long bones arises early so that growth is ultimately stunted. This group of enzyme defects causes complex metabolic changes, which may be life-threatening in some newborn babies because of loss of adrenal gland hormones. They are treated with hormone replacement therapy (hydrocortisone) and possibly surgical reconstruction in girls to restore female genitalia.

congenital and perinatal cytomegalovirus infection (CMV) cytomegaloviruses (belonging to the herpes group) can often be detected in newborn babies, most of whom remain well. The virus is picked up either across the placenta from an infected mother while the baby is in the womb or during passage through the birth canal. After birth, CMV may be acquired through infected breast milk. About 10 per cent of babies with congenital cytomegalovirus infection are seriously affected. Abnormalities include prematurity, low birth weight, a small head, enlargement of the liver and spleen, jaundice, hearing loss, sight defects and mental impairment. About 30 per cent of infected babies die, and those who survive usually suffer from mental impairment, deafness and sight defects. Babies who acquire a perinatal CMV infection may suffer from any of the symptoms described above. Treatment is mainly supportive and aimed at combatting the symptoms that arise. The virus itself is widespread and difficult to treat, although antiviral drugs may be given in some cases.

congenital dermal sinus a deformity present at birth in which there is a channel from the surface of the back to the canal of the spinal cord.

congenital glaucoma, buphthalmos, infantile glaucoma *or* **hydroph-thalmos** a rare CONGENITAL obstruction of fluid (aqueous humour) drainage in the eyes of a newborn baby. If left untreated, it causes a dangerous build-up of fluid and pressure, irreversible damage to the optic nerves and blindness. There is enlargement and bulging of the eyeball and other changes, and usually both eyes are affected. The eyes of a baby should be monitored during the newborn period so that surgery can be carried out at an early stage to prevent any damage.

congenital goitre a CONGENITAL enlargement of the thyroid gland, of which there are four different types, each of which may be accompanied by hypothyroidism (underactivity of the gland). These conditions are associated with defects in the utilisation of iodine and may involve enzyme deficiencies in the production of thyroid hormones (thyroxine). Treatment may involve hormone replacement therapy.

congenital hip dislocation a CONGENITAL abnormality of the hip in which the socket of the joint (acetabulum) is too shallow to accommodate the head of the thigh bone (femur).

congenital hypothyroidism hypothyroidism describes a condition in which there is a lack of the hormone thyroxine that is essential for normal development and growth and is produced by the thyroid gland. The condition is termed congenital hypothyroidism when it is present at birth and in developed countries all newborn babies are tested for the disorder by means of analysing a 'heel-prick' blood sample. About 1 in every 3,500 babies has congenital hypothyroidism and the condition is more common in girls. If the blood test raises suspicions of the existence of the condition, the infant usually undergoes a neck scan to check for the presence of the thyroid gland. Congenital hypothyroidism is usually caused either by the absence of the gland or its displacement to a site where it is unable to function correctly. During foetal development, the thyroid grows at the back of the tongue and later migrates to the neck but in some babies, this process fails to occur. In very rare cases, the gland is correctly sited but is unable to produce thyroxine. In these instances, there is a risk that any future babies born to the parents may be similarly affected.

Usually, congenital hypothyroidism is diagnosed before any symptoms have time to develop but if present, they may include jaundice, sleepiness, difficulty in feeding and constipation. In the absence of treatment there is intellectual and developmental impairment but affected infants are given hormone replacement therapy in the form of thyroxine as a preventative. Most children then develop normally but they require regular check-ups to ensure that they are receiving the appropriate dose of the hormone. In rare cases, hearing can be affected and so periodic testing may be required. A minority of children may continue to experience some degree of learning difficulty, deafness or clumsiness despite treatment but this is uncommon.

congenital kidney defects *see* KIDNEY DEFECTS.

congenital nephroblastoma *see* WILM'S TUMOUR.

congenital non-spherocytic haemolytic anaemia a rare group of disorders involving the processing of red blood cells in which one of several essential enzymes is absent. The lack of enzyme causes haemolytic anaemia in an affected newborn baby, which may vary in severity and requires specialised treatment.

congenital pulmonary arteriovenous fistula an uncommon CONGENITAL abnormality in which there are one or more communicating channels between the arterial (oxygenated) and venous (deoxygenated) blood vessels in the lung. This results in some deoxygenated blood being pumped around the body, and treatment is by means of surgical repair.

congenital scoliosis a CONGENITAL defect of some vertebrae that may also involve certain ribs. It causes abnormal curving of the spine.

congenital syphilis syphilis contracted by a FOETUS across the placenta from an infected mother. In 99 per cent of cases, treatment of the mother with antibiotics during pregnancy brings about a cure and protects the baby. A baby may still acquire the infection if a mother fails to seek adequate medical treatment. Symptoms may appear soon after birth, in which case the condition is known as early congenital syphilis. They include skin lesions, enlarged liver, spleen and lymph glands, failure to thrive, bone changes, MENINGITIS, fits and HYDROCEPHALUS. In other children, the infection may remain dormant until a much later stage or fail to produce any symptoms. If these do arise, they may include skin lesions and ulcers in the mouth and nasal passages, bone changes and neurological disorders, possibly blindness and deafness. Treatment for syphilis is by means of forms of penicillin.

congenital toxoplasmosis toxoplasmosis is an illness caused by a parasitic protozoan micro-organism called *Toxoplasma gondii*. The organism is common throughout the world, affecting about 8 per cent of human populations. Toxoplasma are transmitted by humans eating under-cooked meat containing cysts of the parasite, or by ingesting its eggs, which are present in soil contaminated with infected cat faeces. The organism undergoes sexual reproduction in cats, the eggs passing out in faeces. In other animals and birds, it reproduces asexually within the cells of its host and may form cysts. The host's immune system attacks the organism and renders it ineffective within a period of weeks or months. Hence acquired toxoplasmosis generally produces few or no symptoms, but the CONGENITAL form, passed from an infected mother to her baby before birth, can be extremely severe or fatal. Symptoms may be present at birth or arise shortly afterwards, or their onset may be delayed until later in childhood. A baby may be born prematurely, have a low birth weight, suffer from CONVULSIONS, HYDROCEPHALUS, a small head (microcephalus), jaundice, enlarged liver and spleen, inflammation of the lungs and heart and skin rashes. Eye problems, mental retardation and loss of sight and hearing are other manifestations that may be apparent in infancy or develop in later childhood. A baby may be stillborn or miscarried earlier in pregnancy, and there is a risk of death in infants with severe symptoms.

In general, expectant mothers who acquire toxoplasmosis later in pregnancy are more likely to pass on the infection. However, babies who are infected at an early stage are more likely to exhibit severe symptoms. Children identified as having, or being at risk from, congenital toxoplasmosis require ongoing monitoring, even if they appear well during infancy.

Treatment for those exhibiting symptoms is by means of various drugs, including sulphonamides, pyrimethamine, folinic acid and corticosteroids. Preventative measures are in the form of education so that people become aware of the risks. Women trying to conceive or already pregnant should not handle cat litter and should wear gloves when gardening. Personal hygiene in the form of thorough hand-washing is important and any meat eaten should always be thoroughly cooked. The rate of incidence for congenital toxoplasmosis varies between 1 and 8 infected babies for every 1,000 births, depending on the part of the world involved. In the UK, it has been found that cats now outnumber dogs in popularity as pets and, in addition, there are enormous numbers of feral, stray animals. Inevitably, many of these cats harbour *Toxoplasma gondii* and both the potential for humans to become infected and the risk to unborn children remain high.

conjoined twins identical twins derived from a single fertilised egg who are physically united in one or more regions of the body. In addition to being joined at the skin surface, underlying tissues, nerves, blood vessels and organs may be shared. The separating of conjoined twins is an immensely skilled procedure involving major surgery and possibly more than one operation. One or both infants may not survive.

conjunctivitis neonatorum *see* NEONATAL CONJUNCTIVITIS.

contraception in childhood the idea and the practice of enabling children to have easy access to contraception when they start to become sexually mature is a highly controversial and emotive subject. Most parents readily accept the need for sex education and are happy, and usually relieved, that this is included in the national curriculum. Also, most are concerned about the high number of teenage pregnancies and the apparent degree of ignorance among young people about their own fertility and the prevention of pregnancy. However, the step towards realising that their own son or daughter may be sexually active and in need of contraception, is a giant leap for many parents.

Part of the problem lies in the perceived perception that the boy or girl may become interested in sex at an age when he or she is still very much a child, both legally and in the eyes of parents. Parents are still accustomed to making most of the decisions for their children under 16 years, the legal age for sexual intercourse. However, experience shows that the legal age limit is ineffective in deterring sexual behaviour in adolescents. Many parents are strongly opposed to the idea that their child might receive contraceptive advice without their knowledge or consent, fearing that this might in itself encourage indulgence in sex.

More often than not, however, young people want confidential advice and are reluctant to involve their parents. Studies have shown that the provision of confidential advice and contraception is effective in reducing the incidence of teenage pregnancy. If young people are determined to engage in sexual activity, it is obviously preferable that they should receive thorough counselling and access to contraception. They need to be encouraged to practise 'safe sex', i.e. the use of condoms to lessen the risk of being infected with sexually transmitted diseases or HIV. Girls need to be protected against the possibility of pregnancy, either by means of the contraceptive pill or by hormonal implants. Young people, particularly girls, should be told that there are health risks associated with early sexual activity and should be informed about the need for cervical smear tests to protect against CANCER. In many cases, especially if the child comes from a loving and caring home, it is preferable for parents to be involved but most experts believe that this can only be encouraged and not forced.

convulsions, fits *or* **seizures** involuntary, alternate, rapid muscular contractions and relaxations throwing the body and limbs into contortions. They are caused by a disturbance of brain function and in adults usually result from epilepsy. In babies and young children they occur quite often but, although alarming, are generally not severe. Convulsions are believed to be more common in the very young because the nervous system is immature.

Causes include breath-holding, which is relatively common in infancy or high FEVER as a result of infection or other brain disorder. Emergency medical help should always be summoned if a child has a convulsion so that the underlying cause can be investigated and treated. Usually, the child requires admittance to hospital for a period of observation and/or treatment, depending on the cause of the fit. Convulsions can be a sign of a serious infection such as ENCEPHALITIS or MENINGITIS, but this is not commonly the case.

Cornelia de Lange syndrome a rare congenital disorder of unknown cause affecting about 1 in every 40,000 newborn babies with about 38 new cases each year being reported in the UK. Affected babies are small at birth and continue to be undersized throughout childhood. They have a characteristic appearance with features that include ears set low down, teeth with gaps between them, turned-down lips, snub, up-turned nose, eyebrows that meet centrally over the bridge of the nose and unusually long eyelashes. Abnormalities of the limbs are a common feature such as absence of forearms and affected children are quite often subject to fits. Variable degrees of learning difficulty, ranging from mild to severe, are another characteristic feature. It is believed that the condition is caused by a sporadic mutation in an as yet unidentified gene. Treatment is aimed at relieving accompanying disabilities and ranges from medication to fitting of prosthetic limbs to educational/learning support.

coronary arteriovenous fistula a rare CONGENITAL defect in which there is an abnormal channel between one of the coronary arteries (generally the right) and the right side of the heart, or with a vena cava (one of two major veins returning blood to the heart). Treatment is in the form of corrective surgery.

coronary artery fistula an unusual CONGENITAL defect in which there is an abnormal channel between one of the coronary arteries and the right atrium, ventricle or pulmonary artery. The condition requires corrective surgery.

Costello syndrome *or* **faciocutaneoskeletal syndrome (FCS)** a very rare, inherited condition that produces a range of physical anomalies, a typical pattern of growth and learning disabilities. Affected infants are often large at birth and may have been notably inactive while still in the womb where they are surrounded by an abnormally large quantity of fluid. Other features include a characteristic facial appearance with thick lips, a wide mouth, flattened nose with widely-spaced nostrils, fleshy ear lobes and low-set ears, droopy eye lids and a squint. Children are typically short and curly-haired with bones that are slow to mature. They frequently have loose, stretchy, pigmented skin with small growths around the nose and mouth. Heart problems are commonly present as are difficulties with feeding and there may also be a greater susceptibility to develop certain types of CANCER.

The cause is a mutation in a particular gene (designated HRAS) and there is generally no previous family history of the disorder. A genetic test is now available for Costello syndrome. Treatment takes the form of alleviating the many associated symptoms and problems that can accompany the disorder. It is wide-ranging and can include anything from heart surgery to opthalmology to educational support.

cot death *or* **sudden infant death syndrome (SIDS)** the sudden death of an apparently healthy baby, usually occurring overnight, for which no identifiable cause is subsequently found. The risks are greater in young infants, particularly if the parents smoke, with more boys being affected than girls. Numerous suggestions as to the cause have been put forward. These include viral infections, metabolic respiratory abnormalities, genetic factors and allergic reactions. It is possible that a combination of factors may be involved in each individual case. Cot death is more likely to occur in a baby who has recently had a minor upper respiratory tract infection or other slight ailment. Recently, the sleeping position of the baby has been found to be important in lessening the risk of sudden infant death. The baby should be placed on his or her back, and not on the front or side, when being settled for the night. It is also important not to overwrap the baby – coverings should be light and warm but not too hot.

coughs and colds common, mild infections of the upper respiratory tract caused by viruses. In general, cold symptoms appear first, and these include feverishness, runny nose, sneezing, sore throat, headache and malaise. Children may complain of a feeling of heaviness, loss of appetite or be unusually tired. A cough may become more prominent as other symptoms subside and can be particularly troublesome at night. It may persist for two or three weeks after the initial cold symptoms have improved.

Many children seem to catch one cold after another, particularly when they first begin mixing with friends or start school.

Although this can be a nuisance, the child's natural immunity is built up and strengthened in this way. Most children recover from a cold quickly, and the most that is required is to keep them off school for a day or two if they feel particularly unwell. If a cough is very troublesome and persistent, however, the child should be seen by the family doctor in case a secondary bacterial infection is present that may require antibiotic treatment.

CPD *see* CHILDHOOD POLYCYSTIC KIDNEY DISEASE.

crack cocaine *see* DRUG ABUSE.

cradlecap a common form of seborrhoea or dermatitis of the scalp in young babies in which there is the formation of yellowish crusts. It responds to special shampoos and ointment containing white soft paraffin, salicylic acid and sulphur.

craniopharyngioma a CONGENITAL tumour of the pituitary gland that usually becomes apparent during childhood. It causes disruption of pituitary gland functions and, possibly, HYDROCEPHALUS.

craniostosis (*also* **craniostenosis**) a CONGENITAL abnormality of the skull in which the sutures (the joints between the bones) close prematurely and become ossified, i.e. changed into bone. Growth of the skull is restricted, leading to deformity of the head and pressure on the brain. Surgery is needed to prevent this from occurring, and the condition often occurs in conjunction with other bone abnormalities.

craniosynositosis *or* **Couzon syndrome** a rare, inherited genetic condition affecting about 1 in every 60,000 newborn babies. It is caused by a mutation in a gene that controls a type of growth factor that plays a critical role in the development of skin, bone and connective tissue. Affected children have a characteristic facial appearance due to early fusion of the bones of the skull. Features include a high forehead, beaked nose, abnormally positioned eyes and a small upper jaw and lip. Hydrocephalus with pressure on the brain, deafness, breathing difficulties and skin abnormalities

61

are commonly present. Surgery performed early in life is often needed to release the skull bones, along with insertion of a shunt to drain off fluid and treat the hydrocephalus. Other specialised treatments may also be necessary, depending upon the physical problems that are present and children are likely to require ongoing educational/learning support. In half of all cases, the abnormality arises in the father's sperm and there is an increased risk associated with older fathers. However, in half of all cases there is no previous family history of Couzon syndrome.

crossed eyes *see* STRABISMUS.

croup a symptom caused by a group of diseases affecting young children, characterised by infection, swelling and partial obstruction and inflammation of the entrance to the larynx. Formerly, DIPHTHERIA was the most common cause of croup, but it now usually results from a viral infection of the respiratory tract (laryngotracheobronchitis). Less commonly, a bacterial infection may be the cause. Symptoms are harsh, strained breathing, producing a characteristic crowing sound, accompanying a COUGH and FEVER. There may be pains in the chest and throat, and the child is generally restless and unwell. Attacks may occur at any time but tend to be worse at night. A doctor should be consulted if a child is exhibiting symptoms of croup, but most children can be treated at home. Less commonly, a child may experience severe difficulties in breathing, and this is an emergency that requires immediate medical attention in hospital.

Mild croup can be relieved by creating a steamy atmosphere, e.g. by boiling a kettle or by running hot water into the bath. Also, it is helpful if the child can be persuaded to inhale steam from a bowl or basin of very hot water to which a soothing preparation such as tincture of benzoin may be added. This old-fashioned remedy of sitting with the head bent over a bowl of steaming water enclosed in a 'tent' made from a towel is one of the most effective ways of relieving respiratory discomfort. In addition, mild sedatives and/or painkillers may be advised by the doctor, and the child should be encouraged to drink plenty of fluids. In the rare cases where the obstruction of the throat is severe, the child is treated by nasotracheal intubation or an emergency tracheostomy to restore the airway. Parents should always summon the doctor if the child's breathing starts to become laboured or there are signs of CYANOSIS. Most children make a good recovery from croup, although the condition has a tendency to recur. The child should be discouraged from being out of doors in cold, damp weather as in some cases this may trigger an attack. Likewise, smoking worsens croupy conditions and adults should protect children's health by refraining from this habit.

cryptorchidism a fairly common condition in baby boys in which one of the (or rarely both) testicles fail to descend from the abdomen into the scrotum during development. The condition is corrected by surgery (ORCHIDOPEXY) performed at a young age, in which the testicle is brought down and secured into its correct place in the scrotal sac.

cyanosis a blue appearance of the skin and mucous membranes caused by insufficient oxygen within the blood. It is first noticeable on the lips, tips of the ears, cheeks and nails, and in children occurs where there are breathing difficulties, ASPHYXIA, lung disorders and severe CONGENITAL heart defects (*see* BLUE BABY).

cystinuria an inherited abnormality of the kidneys in which an AMINO ACID called cystine fails to be processed and reabsorbed into the blood. This leads to an elevated amount being present in urine, where it may crystallise to form 'gravel' or stones that may obstruct the urinary tract and increase the likelihood of infections. In addition, the processing of some other amino acids is also reduced, and although these do not precipitate out in the urine, there may be adverse metabolic effects within the body. The condition usually appears in childhood about the age of 10 years, although it may be delayed and occur in young adulthood. Symptoms include kidney pain (renal colic) with the possible development of urinary tract infection.

Treatment consists of increasing fluid intake, especially at night, and taking doses of sodium bicarbonate to make urine more alkaline. Various drugs may also be prescribed. In the long term, sufferers may develop severe complications, including kidney failure.

cystic fibrosis (CF) an inherited (genetic) disease of childhood that affects about one child in every 2000. The defective gene responsible is located on human chromosome 7, and it is quite common within the population, many people being carriers of the abnormality without necessarily being affected themselves. Children of both sexes may inherit cystic fibrosis, and the disease affects all the mucus-secreting glands of the lungs, pancreas, mouth and gastrointestinal tract, and also the sweat glands of the skin. A thick mucus is produced that affects the production of pancreatic enzymes and causes the bronchi to widen (*bronchiectasis*) and become clogged. The child has a constant, severe COUGH, but the mucus is thick and difficult to dislodge. Respiratory infections are common. The stools contain a lot of mucus and are slimy with a foul smell. The child loses weight, and the sweat contains abnormally high levels of sodium and chloride. The liver and spleen become enlarged. The diagnosis of cystic fibrosis is usually made early in the child's life by analysis of the stools, but there is no antenatal test that can detect the condition.

Although cystic fibrosis is incurable, the outlook for affected children has greatly improved, with increasing numbers surviving into adult life. Treatment involves physiotherapy to relieve the bronchial congestion, particularly daily postural drainage, which can be taught to parents so that it can be carried out at home. Humidifiers may be needed in the home to keep the air moist as this helps to thin the mucus. Any respiratory infections should be treated promptly by means of antibiotics. The child may require a special diet that is high in protein and low in fat, along with vitamin supplements and enzyme tablets (to replace pancreatic enzymes). The child may need frequent stays in hospital for intensive nursing care during infections. However, the prognosis is best if he or she is encouraged to lead as active and normal a life as is possible within the limits imposed by the condition. Genetic counselling is normally offered to prospective parents who have a family history of cystic fibrosis so that informed choices can be made about whether to have children.

cystic lymphangioma a cyst composed of lymph tissue that is usually located in the neck, armpit or groin of a child and may be present at birth.

cystinosis a very rare, recessive, inherited disorder in which both parents carry the faulty gene while being unaffected themselves. The gene controls the metabolism of an amino acid called cystine which, in this disorder, abnormally accumulates in cells causing a number of severe problems. There are three types of this disorder: infantile or nephropathic cystinosis, arising during the first year of life; late-onset cystinosis, arising in young people aged 12 years to mid-20s; benign cystinosis, a far less severe form of disorder. The most significant feature of both the infantile and late-onset forms is the accompanying, serious kidney disorder known as Fanconi's syndrome, which leads to kidney failure. Additionally, in infantile cystinosis, there is poor growth, muscle wastage, sight problems and possible blindness, pancreatic damage and diabetes and sometimes, hypothyroidism. Affected children require intensive treatments, drug therapy and special diets. Kidney dialysis and organ transplant are likely to be needed at some stage.

D

Daltonism *see* COLOUR BLINDNESS.

deafness, congenital a partial or complete loss of hearing present at birth may result from a number of conditions, diseases or infections. In the past, GERMAN MEASLES (rubella) was a significant cause of deafness in babies but vaccination has reduced the incidence. Other causes include bleeding within the skull from birth trauma, oxygen deprivation during labour, CONGENITAL TOXOPLASMOSIS and various inherited genetic abnormalities. Special help and education need to be given to a deaf child, beginning in infancy, so that language and communication skills can be acquired. In some cases, the use of highly advanced hearing aids may help.

deciduous teeth, milk teeth *or* **first teeth** the 'baby teeth', which erupt around the age of six months to two years. There are 20 teeth, consisting of four upper and lower incisors (which appear first), two upper and lower canines and four upper and lower molars. Premolars are not present. Deciduous teeth start to be shed at around the age of six years, beginning with the incisors, and have usually all been lost by the age of about 13. They are replaced with a larger number (up to 32) of permanent teeth, which include premolars and the so-called 'wisdom' teeth, that generally do not erupt until about the age of 18 to 20 and may remain within the jaw. (*See* TEETHING.)

dehydration the removal of water. Medically, the loss of water from the body, through sweating, urination, VOMITING and DIARRHOEA during illness which is not replaced by drinking. The person may be too ill to drink or, alternatively, dehydration may arise because there is not water available. Dehydration can arise quite quickly in infants and children as a result of gastrointestinal or feverish illnesses. It is a dangerous condition, which may soon become life-threatening if appropriate treatment is not given, since the salts/water balance is disturbed, causing severe metabolic effects. Signs of dehydration in infants and young children include sunken fontanelle and eyes, hot, dry, flushed skin which loses its elasticity, and crying. Medical help should always be sought if a child shows signs of dehydration or is suffering from repeated diarrhoea and vomiting. The child will often require admittance to hospital for fluid and electrolyte replacement given intravenously, and for treatment of the causal illness.

dental decay *or* **caries** the process by which the surface of a tooth degenerates and crumbles as a result of the formation of plaque (a deposit harbouring bacteria) and bacterial breakdown of sugars and starches in food. The bacterial action results in the formation of acid which dissolves the enamel of the tooth. If not treated, the bacteria are then able to gain access to the deeper layers of the tooth and the infection may eventually result in the formation of a painful abscess. In the United Kingdom, dental decay is a serious problem among infants and children because of the high consumption of sugary foods. Many children have fillings or even extractions of their first teeth before the age of five. Fluoridation of drinking water or giving fluoride drops, thorough cleaning of teeth after meals and before bedtime and, above all, restricting sugary foods and drinks, are all measures that help. Children should also be taken for regular dental check-ups and be educated about the importance of taking care of their teeth.

depression a psychological disorder encompassing feelings of despair, hopelessness, overwhelming sadness and lack of self-worth. Depression used to be considered solely an adult condition but it is now recognised that even quite young children can be affected. It is estimated that about 2 per cent of children aged less than 12 years may suffer from depression with the figure rising to 5 per cent for teenagers. There are a wide range of indications including sadness, listlessness and apathy, loss of interest in friends, hobbies and/or sports, decline in school performance and frequent expression of negative feelings of worthlessness and irritability as well as weight changes, hyperactivity and suicidal thoughts or showing interest in suicide. Physical symptoms may include headaches, stomach and other pains and tiredness. There can be many triggers or causes of depression in children, including bereavement, family break-up, other types of emotional stress, anxiety over exams or school work, bullying, abuse, loss of a close friend, boyfriend or girlfriend. It is very important that adults involved with the child take signs seriously, especially if the young person has ever raised the topic of suicide. The child needs to be encouraged to discuss his or her feelings with a trusted adult, however painful doing this may seem to be. This may need to be with an unconnected adult such as a trained counsellor or psychotherapist. Talking therapies form the basis of treatment for depression in children but occasionally, there may be a need for antidepressant medication. While children usually show a good response to treatment, relapse is fairly common and so ongoing help may be needed for some considerable period of time.

dermatitis a somewhat generalised term for an inflammation of the skin that can have many different causes. If it is an allergic reaction, it is usually called ECZEMA. Symptoms are a reddened, itchy skin that may form small blisters. Contact dermatitis results from contact between the skin and an irritant substance and is a common condition in infancy and childhood. Soaps or detergents and fabric softeners adhering to clothes are frequently implicated, as are fibres in clothing, e.g. wool, which may cause dermatitis, particularly against a child's sensitive skin. Nappy rash is a form of contact dermatitis caused by ammonia in urine. Children may also suffer from light dermatitis caused by a sensitivity to sunlight. The first line of treatment is to remove the cause of the dermatitis. Calamine lotion may relieve mild dermatitis but a child may also need treatment with a topical corticosteroid which must be prescribed by a doctor and used sparingly.

dermatomyositis *see* POLYMYOSITIS.

developmental disorder any one of several conditions in which a normal psychological or intellectual faculty is disrupted. Pervasive developmental disorders involve many functions whereas specific disorders are associated with one only. (*See* AUTISM and DYSLEXIA.)

diabetes *or* **type 1 diabetes** formerly insulin-dependent diabetes mellitus (IDDM) or diabetes mellitus and also called juvenile onset diabetes, brittle diabetes or ketosis-prone diabetes, this is the fairly severe form of diabetes that affects children. It arises because the body is unable to break down sugar and starches in food because of a lack of the hormone insulin. Insulin is normally secreted by the pancreas, an organ in the abdomen that produces digestive juices. Insulin-dependent diabetes tends to arise quite suddenly, and symptoms include excessive thirst and urination, increased appetite but with loss of weight, fatigue and irritability. The condition has to be carefully managed on a long-term basis as this form of diabetes tends to be relatively sensitive and unstable. Treatment is by means of daily insulin injections and control of the diet.

Usually, the child is admitted to hospital in the first instance so that his or her condition can be brought under control and education and support given to the patient and family. Continuing vigilance is needed to avoid ketoacidosis, in which there is an accumulation of ketones in the body along with acidosis (an abnormally high level of acidity in the blood and body fluids). Ketones are organic compounds produced by the liver when fats, rather than carbohydrates, are metabolised to produce energy, as in diabetes when insulin is lacking. Symptoms of ketoacidosis are a fruity 'pear drops' smell on the breath and in urine, confusion and possibly CONVULSIONS, and coma and death if not promptly treated. An immediate injection of insulin is required and possibly intravenous fluids and electrolytes. It is usually necessary for a child to eat regular, small quantities of food to ensure that there is enough glucose in the blood for the amount of insulin given by injection. Missing a meal can lead to the development of hypoglycaemia (too low a level of glucose in the blood) with symptoms of weakness, sweating, and light-headedness, and possibly coma and death if not treated. The condition is alleviated by taking in glucose, either by mouth or by injection if necessary. Childhood type 1 diabetes can be a worrying condition and is one that may be becoming more common. However, with care and positive support, most children become adept at managing their illness and are able to lead a full and normal life.

A worrying new trend has recently been highlighted among young people suffering from type 1 diabetes, that of missing out insulin injections in order to lose weight. Doctors have warned that this is an extremely dangerous practice that can result in coma or even death. The term 'diabulimia' has been coined to describe this practice and it has serious long-term health implications for those who carry it out, increasing especially their future risk of heart problems and blindness.

Diamond-Blackfan syndrome a rare, CONGENITAL blood disorder that becomes apparent in the early weeks of life. The baby becomes extremely anaemic because of a lack of immature red blood cells produced by the bone marrow. However, the white blood cells and blood platelets are not affected.

diarrhoea increased frequency and looseness of bowel movements involving the passage of unusually soft, watery faeces. Diarrhoea is a symptom of many childhood ailments and, if severe, can rapidly lead to DEHYDRATION. Hence a child suffering from persistent diarrhoea should always be seen by a doctor (*see also* ACUTE INFECTIOUS GASTROENTERITIS).

diet a nourishing, well-balanced diet for children is obtained by giving a wide variety of foods containing proteins, carbohydrates, fats, vitamins, minerals and fibre, along with plenty of fluids to drink, preferably water. Children require food both for growth and for what is usually a high level of daily physical activity. Most experts agree that the best foods are those that are eaten in as natural state as possible, i.e. subjected to as little processing and cooking as is safe. However, as most parents soon discover, knowing what constitutes a good diet and persuading their small or adolescent children to eat it are two very different matters! Added to this is the fact that people in the UK are regularly subjected to food scares of one sort or another, so that it can become increasingly difficult and worrying to decide which foods to give. It is also the case that the burden for this usually falls squarely on the mother of the family. In the experience of the author, the best approach is one of good, old-fashioned parental common sense! When children are very small, and particularly with the first-born, it is perfectly possible to give only wholesome foods and to avoid sweets and snacks. It is best to remain calm and unemotional about meals, particularly when a child starts to develop endlessly changing preferences of his or her own, to offer plenty of variety and to remind oneself frequently that one's offspring are unlikely to starve!

As children grow older, they inevitably encounter, and usually develop a taste for, at least some of the endless variety of sweets and 'junk' food. It may be best to allow them to have these kinds of foods occasionally to avoid a build-up of resentment. (For example, children who are never allowed any sweets or crisps at home will often try to obtain them from friends at school.) As children grow older, aspects of food and health can be discussed at home, particularly as they are raised by the media. There is no harm in pointing out that it is sensible to profit from the advice offered by medical experts in relation to diet and in the prevention of diseases such as CANCER. This includes the recommendation to eat at least five portions of fruit and vegetables each day and to choose wholemeal bread, pasta, cereals and rice.

It is also important to lead by example and for children to see that their parents eat a healthy diet. Young children should never be placed on a slimming diet, except in very unusual circumstances and under medical advice. Also, low-fat milk, etc, is inappropriate for this age group as active, growing children need a proportion of fat in their diet. This remains true during the period of rapid growth in the teenage years. Health problems arise only if the child's intake of fat is too high (as is obviously the case in a teenager existing mainly on chips and junk food) and he or she is not taking any physical exercise. Parents should also be aware of the fact that older children, particularly girls, experience considerable social pressures to be slim and may be inclined to eat inadequately at this stage (*see also* ANOREXIA; EXERCISE; OBESITY).

diphtheria a highly contagious bacterial throat infection that is now extremely rare in Western countries. It is caused by the bacterium *Corynebacterium diphtheriae*, and there is the characteristic formation of a fine film or membrane in the throat that can seriously affect breathing. Early symptoms include a sore throat, FEVER, swollen neck glands and pus-filled white spots on the tonsils. The toxins produced by the bacteria can cause severe damage to the heart, kidneys and central nervous system. Hospital admission and isolation are required and treatment with antitoxin, antibiotics and, possibly, tracheostomy (an incision in the trachea or windpipe) to restore the airway. All children in the UK are offered immunisation against diphtheria, and this has proved effective in preventing outbreaks and the fatalities that once occurred.

diphtheria, tetanus toxoids and pertussis vaccine (DTP) a

combined vaccine offered to children in their first year of life
to protect against DIPHTHERIA, TETANUS and WHOOPING COUGH.
Diphtheria and tetanus toxoids vaccination is sometimes given
alone.

discipline is all the means by which parents and other adults teach
children to exercise self-control so that they can learn to behave in
a manner that is acceptable both at home and in the wider world.
The aim is gradually to transform a baby or small child who is
naturally undisciplined into a person who is self-disciplined, i.e.
one who is able to see that his or her desires cannot always come
first or override the needs and feelings of others. The means by
which this should be achieved have become immensely controversial in recent years and are matters that are very much on the
agenda of the United Kingdom government. However, in the
exercise of discipline, either in the home, school or society, there
should be no place for heavy-handed methods that bully children
into submission. It is widely acknowledged that there is also a
greater chance of success if a child is part of a family in which he
or she is loved unconditionally, feels secure and in which there
is an adherence to socially acceptable behaviour. Sadly, for some
children this is not the case.

There has been a fashion among some modern parents to ques-
tion the need to set limits on a child's behaviour, other than
those necessary for ensuring safety. This accompanied a generally
more self-centred outlook, in which the, at times, selfish pursuit
of personal happiness and fulfilment was given a high priority.
However, failing to exercise discipline is doing the child a great
disservice for two reasons. Firstly, children feel happier and more
secure if they know that there are boundaries or limits on their
behaviour beyond which they should not go. Secondly, an undisciplined child is badly behaved and hence unpopular with other
children and adults, and is more likely to feel lonely and isolated,
probably not knowing the reason for this.

The means by which children should be disciplined has been the subject of much debate among child psychologists and parents and in society in general. Most of the many books on childcare offer useful advice on this subject, but parents should also take into account that they themselves are experts and know their own children best. Children are all individuals, and what works for one may be less of a success with another. Also, of course, the methods of discipline should evolve continually as the child matures, and patience, discussion and flexibility are needed!

The most controversial aspect of discipline is whether or not parents should smack their small child as a means of correction. Those who wish smacking to be banned may see no difference between the beating of a child and a parental slap, often delivered in the heat of the moment, merely viewing them as being at either end of a spectrum of physical assault. Interestingly, some of the most fervent advocates of a no-smacking policy admit to having occasionally slapped their own, now usually adult, children when they were young. At the present time, there are no plans in the UK to make it illegal for a parent to smack a child as a means of discipline. It is generally agreed that, if given, a smack should be a last resort and delivered as a light slap on the child's bottom or hand. It should be given at the time of the bad behaviour, and not saved as a punishment for later.

disintegrative psychosis a number of severe disorders that usually appear sometime after the age of three years. The child apparently develops normally until the appearance of the disorder, acquiring language, intellectual and social skills appropriate to his age. The onset of the disorder is usually marked by behavioural changes and irritability, followed by mental deterioration and a loss of all acquired skills. The child ends up severely retarded and, although sometimes a neurodegenerative condition can be found, in other cases the causes remain unidentified. Unfortunately there is no treatment or means of reversing the deterioration and the child requires supportive care for life.

dizygotic twins, non-identical twins *or* **fraternal twins** twins born at the same time as a result of one pregnancy but developed from the union of two different eggs and sperm. Usually only one ovum or egg is released from an ovary each month. If two are released and fertilised then dizygotic twins can develop. Each foetus has its own distinct genetic make-up and may be either male or female, and develops within its own amniotic sac, nourished by a separate placenta. The children may show some similarities as is normal between siblings but are not identical.

Down's syndrome a CONGENITAL chromosomal defect that is usually caused by the presence of an extra chromosome 21, so that there are 47 chromosomes in each body cell instead of the normal 46. At birth, a Down's baby is often floppy, because of poor muscle tone, and of low birth weight with a small, broad head. Characteristic physical features include a broad, round face and flattened nose, slanting eyes (once called 'mongolism') and a large tongue that may protrude. The hands and fingers, feet and toes are short, broad and stubby, and the person is of short stature with weak muscles. There is a degree of intellectual impairment, which varies enormously between individuals. Also, many Down's children have congenital heart defects and respiratory problems, resulting in a high mortality rate in the early years and a generally reduced life expectancy.

In most cases, the extra chromosome originates from the maternal egg, but in about 33 per cent the defect arises in the sperm cell. Other genetic abnormalities cause a rare 3 per cent of cases. Down's syndrome is the most common congenital abnormality, occurring in 1 in every 600 to 800 births. The true incidence may well be higher as it is believed that many affected foetuses are spontaneously aborted in early pregnancy. Until quite recently, Down's syndrome children were unlikely to survive into adulthood, and they were confined in institutions with little being expected of them. Fortunately, the attitude is now much more enlightened and the treatment of those affected has undergone a radical change. It is now recognised that Down's syndrome children vary greatly in their intellectual ability and, given the correct stimulation, support and encouragement, can make very good progress. Special early stimulation, nursery and mainstream education are becoming much more widely accepted, with decisions being made on an individual basis in the best interests of the child. Some severely affected children still need care in a special unit, and others may require extra help with ordinary skills. In adulthood, many Down's syndrome people can lead a fairly independent life in their community, especially with some degree of support.

The incidence of Down's syndrome is strongly correlated with maternal age, changing from 1 in 2,000 births at age 20 to one in 100 at age 40. The cause is not fully understood, but it seems that a woman's eggs are adversely affected by ageing. The risk of all chromosome abnormalities increases if the mother is aged 35 or older. Hence pregnant women in this age group are usually offered AMNIOCENTESIS to detect these conditions, if they so wish, with the possible option of abortion. Abdominal x-rays, viral epidemics and incidence of infectious hepatitis also appear to be correlated with a greater risk of Down's syndrome.

drowning asphyxiation as a result of water entering the lungs. Each year in the UK, a number of children of all ages lose their lives in drowning accidents. A small child can drown in just one or two inches of water, and must never be left alone in the bath or near any stretch of water, however harmless it may seem. Garden ponds should be securely covered with strong wire mesh netting so that a child is unable to fall in. The same is true of water butts, etc, which can attract the attention of an adventurous child. Older children must be educated and constantly reminded about the dangers of open water. All too often, a child is over-confident about his or her swimming abilities or gets cramp because the water is deep and cold. In other cases there may be unforeseen underwater hazards, such as weed or debris in which a child becomes entangled.

A child who has been submerged for more than a few minutes is usually pulled from the water unconscious, showing no pulse or breathing and with a blue coloration of the skin. Emergency treatment must begin immediately, with a check with the fingers to remove any obstacles from the mouth. Artificial respiration and external cardiac massage (cardiopulmonary resuscitation or CPR) should be started at once and the emergency services summoned. Periodic checks should be made for restoration of pulse and breathing, but the CPR should continue until professional help arrives. If the child responds and starts to breathe unaided, he or she should be placed in the recovery position and covered with coats or blankets to keep him or her warm. It is known that a primitive reflex can come into operation in some cases of drowning so that, rarely, even those who have been submerged for some time can be saved.

drug abuse the misuse of a mood-changing substance for its effects, which may cause death or addiction. The term generally refers to illegal substances, and large numbers of teenagers and even younger children admit to having sampled at least one type of drug. An enormous effort is being made in all secondary schools to try to combat the problem and educate children about the very real dangers of taking drugs. The substances that are most likely to be tried by school-age children are solvents, CANNABIS, Ecstasy, possibly amphetamines and tranquillisers, and ALCOHOL and SMOKING. Other drugs, such as heroin, may well be encountered, particularly in areas with a known drug problem. Experimentation may lead on to the abuse of the so-called hard drugs, including heroin and crack cocaine, in young adult life.

The drugs that are commonly abused are described below.

Solvents

These include a wide range of industrial and household chemicals, such as glues, paint thinners, cleaning fluids and cigarette lighter fuel, which are capable of producing toxic effects if inhaled. Abuse of solvents is a particular problem among adolescent boys, and these products are sniffed and inhaled to produce euphoria, elation and hallucination. Other effects include confusion, sleepiness, slurring of speech and staggering. Even with first-time use there is a risk of death through confusion, coma and asphyxiation caused by inhalation of vomit. Prolonged use damages the brain, liver, kidneys and mucous membranes and tissues of the nasal passages, throat and airways.

Cannabis, marijuana, hashish or hemp

This is derived from the Indian hemp plant from which a thick resin is produced. This is smoked, either alone or with tobacco, to produce feelings of euphoria, relaxation, a perceived slowing down of the passage of time and heightened awareness. It appears not to cause physical or psychological damage or withdrawal symptoms, but some medical experts fear that it may cause depressive illness or exacerbate underlying psychiatric conditions. In addition, there is concern that sampling cannabis may progress to experimentation with 'hard' drugs. (*See also* CANNABIS.)

Ecstasy, 'E' or 3.4 methylenedioxymethamphetamine

Ecstasy is similar chemically and in its effects to amphetamines. This has become one of the most commonly used drugs among teenagers and young adults at raves, concerts and dances. Ecstasy, which is taken in tablet form, produces pleasurable emotional feelings of love, goodwill and euphoria. It raises the heart rate and blood pressure and increases endurance, giving the user the capability of dancing through the night. A major risk is that of DEHYDRATION and heat exhaustion, which can lead to collapse and death. The risk is lessened if plenty of fluids are drunk, rests are taken and over-heating is avoided by wearing 'breathable' fabrics that allow evaporation of sweat, but Ecstasy cannot be termed safe. A number of deaths have occurred, some as a result of taking just one tablet. Victims have died painfully through hepatitis and severe liver damage, kidney and heart failure and extreme elevation of body temperature and CONVULSIONS. The greater the dose of Ecstasy taken at any one time, the higher the risk of damage or death, particularly if the tablets are impure.

Ecstasy tablets are produced illegally for the drug scene and are frequently contaminated with chemicals, amphetamines or LSD. Among the young there is a widespread view that Ecstasy does not produce long-term harm or addiction and that those who have died have been unlucky or failed to take precautions. In fact, medical experts believe that Ecstasy does leave its mark in the form of physical and psychological damage which may not be immediately apparent. A strenuous effort is being made by those who have first-hand knowledge of the devastating effects of Ecstasy to convince young people of the dangers of this drug.

Amphetamines

Amphetamines, or 'speed', are a group of drugs that are chemically similar to the naturally occurring hormone adrenaline and have a marked stimulating effect on the central nervous system. They act on the sympathetic nervous system, producing feelings of supreme mental alertness and increased energy, eliminating tiredness. They were formerly used medically as appetite suppressants in the treatment of OBESITY, but because of their addictive and dangerous nature, this practice has been discontinued. Amphetamines continue to be prescribed in strictly controlled conditions in the treatment of hyperkinetic syndrome, a mental disorder in children. These drugs are sometimes abused by people in situations demanding mental alertness or by those who wish to continue working for a prolonged period. In small amounts, amphetamines raise heartbeat rate and blood pressure and suppress the need for sleep, but they soon produce tolerance so that the user needs to take a larger dose. In these circumstances, or in overdose, blood pressure may rise to dangerous levels and there may be palpitations, hallucinations and, rarely, convulsions. Prolonged abuse leads to dependence, along with paranoia, feelings of persecution and unpredictable aggressive reactions. Amphetamines are occasionally used to counteract the effects of depressants, or 'downers', such as barbiturates, by those who regularly abuse drugs. Their use in these circumstances is especially dangerous.

A more recent development is the spread among young clubbers of the highly addictive synthetic drug known as 'crystal meth' (methamphetamine) which can be smoked, swallowed, snorted or injected. The 'high' produced by this drug can last for 3 to 4 hours but the 'comedown' is severe with feelings of hopelessness and despair. The risks associated with this dangerous stimulant include depression and other mental health problems such as paranoia, severe weight loss, kidney failure, internal bleeding and tooth decay as well as violent and aggressive behaviour.

Sedatives

Sedatives are drugs that lessen tension and anxiety and are hypnotics, i.e. can be used to induce sleep. They have a depressive effect on the central nervous system and may be used medically to control pain, insomnia, spasms, EPILEPSY and extreme anxiety. Examples are barbiturates, which reduce blood pressure and temperature and depress respiration. Prolonged use of these powerful drugs leads to physical and psychological dependence and overdose can cause death as a result of cessation of breathing. If a person has been taking sedatives for some time, the dose must be reduced gradually to avoid the occurrence of withdrawal symptoms.

Tranquillisers

Tranquillisers are central nervous system depressants that, like sedatives, have a soothing and calming effect, relieving stress and anxiety. Minor tranquillisers, including benzodiazepines such as diazepam (Valium) and flurazepam (a hypnotic), are widely used to relieve these symptoms, which may arise from a variety of causes. There is a danger of dependence with use exceeding a period of one or two weeks so they are now generally prescribed for short-term relief. In the past, tranquillisers were over-used because patients became dependent on them, continuing to take them long after the original need had declined. Falsification of prescriptions and other devious methods enable them to fall into the wrong hands. They may be taken by regular drug abusers as 'downers' to counteract the effects of central nervous system stimulants such as amphetamines. Major tranquillisers, e.g. chlorpromazine and haloperidol, are used to treat severe mental illnesses such as schizophrenia.

Opiates

These are a group of drugs derived from opium. This is a milky liquid extracted from the unripe seed capsules of the poppy, *Papaver somniferum*, which contains almost 10 per cent of anhydrous morphine. Other opiates include heroin, the synthetic derivative of morphine, methadone and codeine. All are central nervous system depressants that are used medically to relieve severe pain and suppress coughing (methadone). They are

81

narcotics, i.e. are capable of producing stupor and loss of awareness. In addition, respiration and the cough reflex are depressed and muscle spasms may be produced. Regular use causes the development of tolerance and dependence, and these drugs are commonly abused, generally by intravenous injection. Heroin is a white crystalline powder, also known as diamorphine hydrochloride, which has various 'street' names and is one of the most common of the 'hard drugs'. It is highly addictive and dangerous, and heroin abusers commonly die young as the result of an accidental overdose or because the drug is 'cut', i.e. mixed with poisonous impurities. A baby born to a mother who uses heroin is severely affected (*see* DRUG-ADDICTED BABY). Heroin abusers are frequently involved in crime to fund their habit and are generally in poor physical condition, with their whole lives revolving around their addiction. There are special clinics to help users to be cured of their addiction, but this can be a hard and painful process that usually succeeds only if self-motivation is very strong.

Cocaine

Cocaine (informally known as 'coke') is an alkaloid substance derived from the leaves of the South American coca plant. It has a rapid and localised effect on mucous membranes and skin, producing anaesthesia, and was formerly much used in nose, throat, ear and eye surgery. However, when absorbed, cocaine causes significant biochemical changes in the brain, having a stimulating effect. It produces intense but relatively short-lived feelings of increased energy, alertness and excitement, raising blood pressure and heartbeat rate. Further doses, particularly in large amounts, can result in death through heart failure, CONVULSIONS or brain haemorrhage or the development of paranoid psychotic states.

The euphoria produced by cocaine has led to the drug being

widely abused, mainly by 'snorting' the powder through the nose, which causes thinning of nasal tissue, bleeding and even perforation of the dividing septum between the nostrils. Regular doses of cocaine produce psychological dependence and strong cravings for its effects, but in between use, addicts commonly experience lethargy and depression. Because of its highly addictive and dangerous nature, cocaine is now infrequently used in medicine, although it may still be prescribed to relieve severe pain in terminal cancer.

Crack cocaine

Crack cocaine is a purified, more potent form of cocaine usually manufactured as small, peanut-sized pebbles that are smoked by means of a water pipe. It produces a stronger, more immediate psychological effect than cocaine, with feelings of intense physical and mental wellbeing. However, these feelings last for only 10 to 15 minutes and are replaced by symptoms of anxiety, depression, appetite loss and insomnia. Users frequently lose weight and develop a wheezing chronic cough and voice changes. Hallucinations, paranoid and bizarre behavioural changes and increased risk of suicide all may accompany prolonged use. Accidental overdose of crack can cause death from heart attack, respiratory failure and CONVULSIONS.

LSD or lysergic acid diethylamide

LSD is one of a group of extremely potent, hallucinogenic drugs, other examples being mescaline and various plant chemicals such as those found in some mushrooms and toadstools. The main feature of LSD is that it produces hallucinations that can be pleasant but more often induce extreme terror. Such is the state of altered consciousness that, under the influence of LSD, people have believed that they are able to fly and have fallen to their deaths from high buildings. The drug has numerous side effects, including changes in behaviour and perception, anxiety, depression, nausea, trembling, visual disturbances, lack of coordination and sweating. Tolerance develops very rapidly, even with small doses, and frightening 'flashbacks' triggered by some external stimulus such as a piece of music can occur when the drug is no longer being used. LSD was formerly used in the treatment of some psychiatric conditions but, because of the dangers associated with it, has now been withdrawn.

Anabolic steroids

These are synthetic male hormones, similar to naturally occurring ANDROGENS, that are used medically to treat conditions requiring increased muscle and tissue growth. These conditions include severe debilitating illnesses, certain growth defects in children, some cases of osteoporosis and renal failure, hypoplastic ANAEMIA, LEUKAEMIA and long-term corticosteroid treatment. All anabolic steroids produce virilising effects to a certain extent (i.e. they promote the development of masculine secondary sexual characteristics), although they are generally less potent in this respect than androgens. In the highly competitive world of sports and athletics, young people can be tempted to abuse anabolic steroids because these substances have the ability to build up muscle mass and strength. This has serious consequences for health, potentially causing liver disease, increased risk of cancer, infertility and effects on the pituitary gland. In all sporting activities, there are regular and rigorously applied on-the-spot checks for abuse of these and other drugs, and those testing positive face bans and disgrace.

The abuse of drugs usually causes altered behaviour, and this is frequently the factor that alerts parents to the fact that their child may be experimenting with them. The young person may be appear to be withdrawn or agitated, with increased sensitivity to sights and sounds, and the use of heroin and cocaine causes the pupils of the eyes to contract to pinpoints. Tackling the problem can be undoubtedly difficult, and professional help is usually needed, probably involving the family doctor, the school and possibly the police. While no parent wishes to see his or her child getting into trouble, drug abuse among young people is a serious problem involving substances that are illegal. Having to face up to the potentially serious social as well as health consequences of drug taking is likely to be a strong discouragement to further experimentation. If the young person has already become addicted to a particular substance, then specialist professional treatment is needed from a drugs clinic.

Understandably, many parents feel out of their depth in even attempting to discuss the issue of drugs with their children. However, many experts believe that it is vital for drugs to be talked about, not only at school but in the home also. It is also crucial for parents to avoid making the mistake of thinking that their own child would never become involved with drugs and to take the time and trouble to become as well informed as possible.

drug-addicted baby drugs that are commonly abused are able to cross the placenta to a developing FOETUS, if taken during pregnancy. This may not only result in physical and neurological damage but also causes the baby to become addicted to the drug. Hence, after birth, the infant suffers from distressing withdrawal symptoms because the accustomed drug dose is no longer available. Withdrawal symptoms in a newborn baby include fretfulness and crying, sickness and DIARRHOEA, rapid breathing, sweating, increased irritability, floppy muscles and CONVULSIONS. Treatment depends on the severity of the symptoms but sedatives such as phenobarbital may be needed. The use of cocaine and crack cocaine (*see* DRUG ABUSE) during pregnancy may cause spontaneous abortion and increased likelihood of the dangerous condition called abruptio placentae in which the placenta can become completely detached. In addition, the baby is of low birth weight and achieves a poor score in tests carried out immediately after delivery (*see* APGAR SCORE). The child may have physical abnormalities of the limbs and digestive tract and brain damage.

DTP *see* DIPHTHERIA, TETANUS TOXOIDS AND PERTUSSIS VACCINE.

duodenal atresia a rare, congenital abnormality of the duodenum which is the first part of the intestine, leading off from the stomach. In duodenal atresia, the tube is blocked so that fluid and food cannot pass into it from the stomach in the normal way. The condition is sometimes diagnosed before birth and babies with this abnormality are often premature. This disorder has a particular association with Down's Syndrome, affecting 33 per cent of children with that condition. A baby with duodenal atresia becomes ill as soon as it starts to feed and the only treatment is surgery, which is performed soon after birth to reinstate the duodenal passageway. Most babies make a full recovery and are soon able to feed normally.

Duchenne muscular dystrophy a wasting disease of the muscles, which is a sex-linked, recessive disorder carried on the X-chromosome. Females can be carriers of the disease but symptoms can only be expressed in males, and they usually first appear in boys aged between three and seven years. The disease causes muscle fibres to degenerate, and usually those of the pelvic girdle (hips) and shoulder girdle are attacked first. Early symptoms include a peculiar, waddling gait, numerous falls, difficulty in standing up and in going down stairs. The spine curves inwards, a condition known as lordosis, and the child walks on his toes rather than placing the heel down first. The muscles appear large and firm, but this is because of the internal changes that are taking place with a build-up of fibrous and fatty tissue. Muscles become progressively weaker, and the child is usually confined to a wheelchair by about the age of 12. There is no specific drug treatment, although clinical trials on the corticosteroid prednisone are being carried out, and the disease is the subject of ongoing research. Therapy is aimed at keeping the child as mentally and physically alert and active as possible, using physiotherapy, massage and orthopaedic measures. Unfortunately, serious life-threatening complications can arise, especially chest and other infections such as pneumonia. Most affected boys develop heart abnormalities.

dwarfism an abnormal underdevelopment of the body manifested by small stature, beginning in childhood. There are a number of different causes, including hormonal defects resulting from incorrect functioning of the pituitary or thyroid gland. Pituitary dwarfism produces a small but correctly proportioned body, and if diagnosed sufficiently early, treatment with synthetic growth hormone can help to correct the defect. A defect in the thyroid gland may result in CRETINISM. Malabsorption disorders involving the digestive system and its secretions are a further cause of dwarfism, as are deficiency diseases such as RICKETS. Modern methods of treatment can usually help to correct these disorders and restore a more normal pattern of growth.

dyskinetic syndrome a condition related to CEREBRAL PALSY involving the basal ganglia of the brain. Symptoms include ATHETOSIS, which is usually more noticeable when the child is tense orexcited. These movements diminish when the child is relaxed or sleeping.

dyslexia (popularly called 'word blindness') a disorder that makes it difficult to learn to read. There is usually an associated problem in writing and spelling words correctly. A small number of children are affected quite severely, and in the past there was a problem in recognising dyslexia so appropriate help was often not given. There is now a much greater awareness of dyslexia, and a child experiencing learning difficulties can be referred for special tests that can diagnose the condition. Special educational methods are needed to overcome the problems posed by dyslexia so that the child can be taught to read. The condition does not in any way denote a lack of intellectual capability but the reasons why it occurs are imperfectly understood.

dysmenorrhoea pain at the time of menstruation, which is an extremely common condition, experienced by most women at some time or other. However, in a few cases the pain can be severe and disabling and may arise in a young girl as soon as she starts to have monthly periods. The pain is spasmodic and cramp-like, often accompanied by nausea, DIARRHOEA and digestive upset, and is usually worse just prior to, or during, the first day or two of menstruation. It usually lasts for several hours or even longer, and the girl is not able to attend school because the symptoms are too severe. In these circumstances, it is necessary for the girl to receive treatment, usually hormonal, to control the symptoms.

dyspraxia a movement and developmental disorder affecting physical and intellectual capabilities and learning. Affected children experience difficulty in mastering normal physical and coordination skills such as running and jumping and they frequently appear as awkward and clumsy. Language skills and speech may be poor and there can be problems in mastering everyday skills such as dressing and brushing teeth. There may be learning difficulties that only become apparent when the child starts school but the disorder affects individuals in different ways. Also, an affected child shows individual inconsistencies in, for example, being able to carry out a task on one day but being unable to repeat it on the next.

All this makes dyspraxia a challenging disorder, not only for the affected child but also for those involved in care and treatment. A whole range of disciplines may be employed to help a dyspraxic child, ranging from speech therapy to learning support and psychotherapy. For reasons that are not clear, boys are at a four-fold greater risk of this disorder. In some cases, a developmental problem in the womb or a lack of oxygen affecting the brain during a difficult birth can be identified as a cause. A brain injury or illness such as *encephalitis* can also be the cause of dyspraxia in a child who was previously well and the condition can sometimes run in families, for reasons that are poorly understood. But in some children, no obvious cause of the dyspraxia can be identified.

E

'E' *see* DRUG ABUSE.

echinococcosis *see* HYDATID CYST.

E coli *see* ESCHERICHIA COLI.

Ecstasy *see* DRUG ABUSE.

eczema an inflammation of the skin, which is usually caused by an allergy and is a form of DERMATITIS. The most common form affecting children is called *infantile* or *atopic eczema*, which usually begins around the age of three to four months but can be earlier or later. Reddening of the skin begins on the scalp and spreads to the face and, in some cases, to other parts of the body. The skin erupts with small, fluid-filled spots that 'weep' and are very itchy, and the child finds it impossible not to scratch. This leads to increased irritation and possibly secondary bacterial infection. Approximately 70 per cent of affected children have a family history of ASTHMA, HAY FEVER or eczema. The application of a steroid cream or ointment such as one containing 1 per cent hydrocortisone may be prescribed and must be used in strict accordance with instructions. In babies and small children, mittens may be needed to cover the hands and prevent scratching, especially during sleep. Rarely, a sedative may be needed to prevent scratching and give the skin a chance to heal. Infantile eczema frequently improves as a child grows older.

Ehlers-Danlos syndrome (EDS) an inherited disorder of connective tissue in which the joints are highly mobile, the skin is unusually elastic and the tissues are very fragile. Scarring is common over joints and the skin is subject to tearing. Various skeletal abnormalities, dislocations and sprains, and also eye disorders, are commonplace. There are a number of different varieties of Ehlers-Danlos syndrome, which may each show particular clinical features. There is no specific treatment but children may benefit from wearing protective, padded clothing to lessen the risk of injury.

embryological development the various stages of development and differentiation undergone by an embryo during the first 8 weeks of life, during which enormous changes take place and in which the embryo is vulnerable to damage.

Emery-Dreifus syndrome an uncommon, recessive genetic disorder carried on the X-chromosome, which affects the joints and the heart and appears in early childhood.

encephalitis, post-infectious encephalitis is inflammation of the brain, which is most commonly caused by a viral infection. Post-infectious encephalitis can arise as a complication of a number of common childhood diseases, including MEASLES and CHICKEN POX. Symptoms include FEVER, headache, neck stiffness, generalised aches and pains, fatigue, weakness and irritability. If the condition worsens, the patient may become disorientated and confused, with CONVULSIONS, paralysis and eventually COMA.

Encephalitis is a serious condition requiring emergency admittance to hospital for intensive treatment and nursing. Death may occur, and there is also a risk of permanent brain damage. Usually the spinal cord is also affected and so the condition is more correctly post-infectious encephalomyelitis. It was a potential cause of death in measles outbreaks before the introduction of vaccination.

endocarditis inflammation of the endocardium, the inner lining of the heart, that is caused by bacterial or viral infection. It usually arises in people with a damaged heart, and in children this damage is normally CONGENITAL. It is rare before the age of five, and treatment is by means of antibiotics and supportive care.

enterobiasis *see* THREADWORMS.

epidemic pleurodynia (Bornholm disease) an infectious illness that is usually caused by one of the coxsackie group of viruses (or echoviruses), affecting the intercostals muscles of the chest and sometimes, the lungs and pleura. It tends to occur in epidemics in the summer and autumn and mainly affects children and young adults. The virus is excreted in faeces and is readily passed on between small children via contamination spread by the fingers onto toys or food items. The symptoms are spasmodic pain varying in intensity, affecting the chest and upper abdominal region and also, pains in the neck and limbs. The infection usually begins with flu-like symptoms, malaise and pains that occur for about 20 to 30 minutes at a time. In children, symptoms generally begin to subside after about two days but they may flare up again around three weeks later.

Treatment involves painkillers and bed rest until the symptoms subside. Immunoglobulin given intravenously may be needed for infants or young children with weakened immunity or who are suffering from some other existing disorder or illness.

epidermolysis bullosa (EB) a group of inherited disorders affecting the skin and mucous membranes in which the defining feature is extreme fragility and blistering. The blisters not only arise on the skin but can occur in the mouth and gastrointestinal tract, causing scarring and contraction. Constipation is a recognised complication, arising because blisters around the anus make passing faeces extremely painful. There are at least 21 known types of EB. Some have a dominant pattern of inheritance (i.e. only one copy of the faulty gene needs to be present for EB to arise) while other types are recessive (two copies of the faulty gene are inherited, one from each parent). In general, forms of EB with a dominant inheritance pattern are less severe. One in every 227 people is a carrier of the faulty gene for EB, but often they are themselves unaffected and healthy. An antenatal test is now able to detect EB between 8 and 10 weeks of pregnancy. About 1 in every 17,000 newborn babies has some form of EB and the condition can arise in both sexes equally. Three types of the disorder predominate: dystrophicEB or DEB, EB simplex or EBS, and junctional EB.

In DEB, there may be extensive scarring resulting from the blisters which can in itself cause considerable disability. Also, DEB may be either dominant (termed DDEB) or recessive (termed RDEB) with the latter showing a range of severity from mild to fatal. EBS almost exclusively shows a dominant pattern of inheritance and there are three main types: Weber-Cockayne, Kobner, and Dowling Meara. Weber-Cockayne is the most prevalent and the distinguishing factor is blisters that arise only on the feet and hands. Sometimes, the blisters on the feet only occur when an infant starts to learn to walk. In Kobner EBS, blisters are usually apparent at birth or in the early weeks of life. They often occur at sites of rubbing such as the nappy area and may also arise in the mouth. Junctional EB, which arises in 10 per cent of those affected, is a very severe form of the disorder in which there is blistering and scarring within the gut. About half of children die during early childhood. All forms of EB require specialist treatment to manage the blisters and any skin wounds that occur. Drug treatments may be needed along with a high-fibre diet to prevent constipation. Special attention has to be given to clothing and footwear, choosing materials and brands that have the least impact upon the skin.

epiglottitis a relatively rare inflammation and swelling of the epiglottis (the cartilage separating the back of the tongue from the entrance to the airway, which closes the latter during swallowing). The condition is most common in children aged one to six years and is caused by a bacterial infection that is rarely spread from child to child. Symptoms include FEVER, noisy, difficult breathing, COUGH, excessive production of saliva and rapid pulse, which arise rapidly over a few hours. Immediate admittance to hospital is needed for treatment with antibiotics. If obstruction to breathing is severe, intubation may be needed (the patient is sedated and a tube inserted into the airway) or, in very serious cases, a tracheostomy (an incision into the trachea) may be performed.

epilepsy *or* **falling sickness** a neurological disorder characterised by the occurrence of CONVULSIONS or seizures and a loss of consciousness or momentary loss of awareness. It usually begins in childhood between the ages of 2 and 14, and quite commonly in children under 5 years old. There are several forms of epilepsy and, characteristically, the symptoms arise quite suddenly. A *petit mal* seizure is common in children and is characterised by a loss of awareness. The child suddenly stops the activity in which he or she is engaged and looks blank, being unaware of his or her surroundings. There may be some odd muscular movements or changes of expression. The attack usually lasts for a very short time and the sufferer then normally comes round and resumes the previous activity, often unaware of the episode.

A *grand mal* seizure may also occur in a child and involves a sudden complete loss of consciousness. The person falls to the ground, the muscles are stiff and he or she has a rapid pulse, pallor and dilated pupils. The body is then thrown into spasms by violent jerking of the muscles. The person may gnash the teeth, bite the tongue and froth at the mouth, and the eyes roll in the head. Breathing is noisy, and there may be loss of control of bowel and bladder function. The attack usually lasts for up to a few minutes and the body then relaxes. Consciousness may be regained to a certain extent but is usually accompanied by confusion, and the person often falls into a deep sleep that may last for a few hours. On waking, the person may feel back to normal or may feel tired, subdued and depressed. Treatment is tailored to each individual's requirements, and various anticonvulsive drugs are used to control epilepsy. The type and dose that is most effective varies between individuals, and a person with epilepsy requires periodic check-ups and monitoring. The condition generally cannot be cured but can be well controlled so that an affected child can generally lead a normal life. There are many possible causes but very often this cannot be discerned in a particular case.

epispadias a CONGENITAL disorder of the urethra that can arise in both sexes but is rare in females. In boys, the urethra opens on the upper surface of the penis instead of at the end, in the region of the glans. Surgical correction is needed but there may be problems of urinary incontinence.

erythema any one of a number of skin conditions characterised by the engorgement of superficial blood vessels and the appearance of red, inflamed patches. Erythema multiformae is most common in children and young people, especially girls. Red blotches, lumps and blisters appear on the hands, arms and body, but symptoms are variable. It is believed to be caused by a virus but also occurs as an allergic response to certain drugs. Erythema infectiosum ('slapped cheek' disease) is a highly contagious condition, caused by a human parvo virus, which usually affects children during the months of spring. A bright red rash appears on the cheeks and spreads to other areas, usually subsiding after about three weeks. Erythema neonatorum is a pink rash that quite commonly arises in newborn babies, occurring on the body and generally subsiding after a few days. Treatment for erythema depends on the type involved and the severity of the symptoms. Various drugs may be used, e.g. corticosteroids and non-steroidal anti-inflammatory preparations, in some cases.

erythroblastosis foetalis an uncommon but severe form of haemolytic anaemia that occasionally arises in a newborn baby because of an incompatibility between foetal and maternal blood. An antibody-ANTIGEN reaction is generated that involves the rhesus and ABO blood antigens. The condition begins before birth when maternal antibodies pass via the placenta to the FOETUS and may result in stillbirth.

erythroedema, erythromelalgia *see* ACRODYNIA.

Escherichia coli *or* **E coli** a group of bacteria that are normally present in the gut, one strain of which has recently emerged to cause serious outbreaks of food poisoning. Illness is particularly severe in young children (and the elderly) and may cause death, or disability in the form of kidney damage in those who survive.

Ewing's sarcoma a rare, very malignant cancer of bone that arises most commonly in children and young people between the ages of 10 and 20 years. It is more common in boys than in girls and usually first affects the limb or pelvic bones. Symptoms include pain, swelling, tenderness, FEVER and a raised white blood cell count. Treatment is by means of radiotherapy and chemotherapy, and surgical amputation of a limb may be necessary in some cases. With localised Ewing's sarcoma, combined therapy is successful in over 60 per cent of cases.

exanthem subitum *see* ROSEOLA INFANTUM.

exercise is needed at all ages to ensure good health, and in childhood it should arise quite naturally through active play. However, there is considerable concern that many children in Britain today have a much less healthy lifestyle than was the case for former generations. This concern centres not only on the fact that many children eat a high-fat, high-sugar diet but also that they have a more sedentary lifestyle. Many children are no longer encouraged to go out to play, especially in the cities, as the environment is perceived to be too dangerous, and now even short journeys are made by car instead of on foot. In addition, the revolution in the choice and sophistication of toys, games, television and computers has meant that there are many absorbing indoor occupations, lessening the attraction of playing outside. For many children, energetic activities are now restricted to organised games and sports at school or occasional family outings to a leisure centre or swimming pool.

It is believed that large numbers of children, especially in the older age groups, are simply too inactive, and many are overweight and will pay the price in adult life in the form of early heart disease. School sports tend to become increasingly unpopular in the teenage years so that many older children take very little exercise at all. It is impossible to lay down hard and fast rules, but it should be remembered that children follow the example set by their parents. It is therefore important to make time for physical activities, which can be something as simple as a trip to the local park, and to encourage children's natural enthusiasm and interest in energetic pursuits and sports as they grow older.

exercise-induced asthma a contraction of the bronchioles (very fine tubes or air passages in the lungs) in an asthmatic child brought about by hard physical exertion. This causes breathlessness and wheezing and arises because the child has highly sensitive and reactive air passages. The condition varies in severity, and in mild cases may be hardly noticed by the child, so that it is to be hoped it can be successfully controlled by medication and exercise need not be restricted. It is more likely to be a problem if the child has a cold or some other infection and hard exertion should be avoided at this time.

Studies carried out in Scotland revealed quite a high incidence of exercise-induced asthma among school children, a number of whom had not previously been identified as being asthmatic. The condition may therefore be more common than is generally realised and may, in some cases, go undetected.

F

Fabry disease a rare, genetic disorder in which there is a lack of the enzyme alpha-galactoside A which is involved in the metabolism of lipids (fats). The defective gene is located on the X-chromosome and hence boys are much more likely to be affected than girls (as their genetic make-up is XY). The enzyme deficiency causes a build-up of certain fats called glycosphingolipids in the tissues and organs, particularly in the kidneys, heart and nervous system. The degree of enzyme deficiency varies considerably and this affects the age at which the condition is manifested. The greater the extent of deficiency the earlier the onset of symptoms. Hence, when children are affected, it usually correlates with a serious lack of the enzyme.

Symptoms include pain and burning sensations, especially in the hands and feet, purplish-red, raised spots (called angiokeratomas) on the skin and inside the mouth, changes inside the cornea and lens of the eyes and a reduced ability to sweat, affecting temperature regulation. There is an increased risk of heart and kidney problems and stroke. Treatment may involve enzyme supplements and other medication to deal with particular symptoms. There is no cure but gene therapy may prove to be effective in the future.

face scanning (a diagnostic aid for genetic disorders) medical research scientists have recently (2007) developed a computerised system to detect the facial anomalies associated with many congenital, genetic disorders. These heart and face syndromes often produce subtle facial differences that can be difficult to detect with any degree of certainty with the naked eye, especially during infancy or early childhood. The new system is able to detect 30 different conditions with a 90 per cent degree of accuracy and is being hailed as a useful tool for early diagnosis. It is believed that prompt diagnosis will help to speed up investigation and treatment of any potentially serious physical and developmental problems that so frequently accompany these rare disorders. The disorders that can be diagnosed by this technique include FRAGILE X SYNDROME, JACOBSEN'S SYNDROME, NOONAN'S SYNDROME, SMITH-MAGENIS SYNDROME and WILLIAM'S SYNDROME.

falling sickness *see* EPILEPSY.

familial iminoglycinuria a benign, recessive condition of the kidneys in which the amino acids proline, hydroxyproline and glycine are excreted in the urine rather than being reabsorbed. It does not require specific treatment.

Fanconi's anaemia a rare CONGENITAL condition in which there is anaemia along with bone and developmental abnormalities.

Feingold diet a dietary regime devised by an American paediatrician, Benjamin Feingold, for the control of hyperactivity in children (*see* ATTENTION DEFICIT DISORDER; HYPERACTIVITY). Permitted foods exclude all artificial additives, and certain fruits and vegetables are also restricted.

fertility, preservation of a possible breakthrough was announced in 2007 by a team of doctors and scientists in Israel that may enable the fertility of young girls who have to undergo aggressive cancer treatments to be preserved. The team have succeeded in harvesting and freezing eggs from the ovaries of girls as young as 5 years of age, prior to the onset of cancer treatment that routinely either destroys or greatly reduces future fertility. The hope is that the eggs can one day be used to produce biological offspring in women whose childhood treatment would usually have left them infertile.

fever *or* **pyrexia** a rise in body temperature above normal, which is, in itself, quite variable but is generally accepted as being 37.4°C orally or 37.6°C rectally. Fever is common in childhood and is primarily caused by viral or bacterial infections but may arise with other diseases, tumours, autoimmune disorders or shock. A fever is a symptom rather than a disease and, at its outset, may be marked by shivering and chills. In addition there may be headache, sickness, thirst, DIARRHOEA or CONSTIPATION, back and joint pains. This is often followed by an increase in pulse and breathing rate, hot, dry, flushed skin, marked thirst and loss of appetite and reduced urination. In young children a fever that rises to above 40.5°C may cause CONVULSIONS and delirium. Antipyretic drugs to lower the temperature, which are suitable for children, are likely to be needed along with sponging the body with tepid water or using cooling fans. The doctor should always be called as it is vital that the underlying cause of the fever is identified so that appropriate treatment may be given.

first teeth *see* DECIDUOUS TEETH.

fits *see* CONVULSIONS.

flat foot *or* **pesplanus** an absence of the arch of the foot so that the inner edge lies flat on the ground. It is common in small children who are just beginning to walk as the ligaments of the foot are soft, but is usually naturally corrected between the ages of two to three years. True CONGENITAL flat-footedness that persists beyond infancy is treated by means of corrective built-up footwear and, possibly, exercises or surgery.

floppy baby syndrome a baby who has little or poor muscle tone at birth, which can arise because of a number of different causes.

focal segmental glomerulosclerosis (FSGS) a kidney disorder affecting the glomeruli – a network of minute tubules that filter the blood passing through the kidneys, allowing waste products to pass out in urine while retaining useful molecules such as proteins. In FSGS, a proportion of the glomeruli become scarred and damaged, so allowing a loss of protein in the urine and the onset of NEPHROTIC SYNDROME. FSGS is more properly a group of disorders, some of which result from certain inherited conditions while others may have an autoimmune origin (one in which the body's immune system attacks its own tissues). But in other instances, the cause of FSGS remains unknown. About 7 to 10 per cent of children with nephrotic syndrome are diagnosed as having FSGS and treatment comprises various drugs including steroids, immunosuppressants, preparations that reduce protein loss and diuretics. FSGS may eventually lead to kidney failure, necessitating dialysis and ultimately, transplant surgery.

food intolerance a condition in which the body is unable to deal with a certain food or food component, usually due to a deficiency in the enzyme that normally metabolises the particular substance involved. The condition can be distinguished from food ALLERGY because it is not an allergic response and does not involve the immune system. There is a strong racial pattern of inheritance of the various known food intolerances, possibly relating to dietary differences among early human populations who were separated geographically from each other. One of the best known food intolerances is lactose intolerance, lactose being a type of sugar found, for example, in cow's milk. It is caused by a deficiency in the enzyme lactase and affected children suffer symptoms such as abdominal cramps, diarrhoea and bloating. However, most babies are born with an excess of lactase gained from their mother and so the symptoms of milk intolerance may not begin immediately. The disorder is usually managed by avoidance of the food group involved and children can be given soya milk or other special formulas, once a diagnosis has been made.

foetal alcohol syndrome a group of CONGENITAL abnormalities caused by maternal intake of ALCOHOL during pregnancy, which vary in severity depending on the level consumed. In severe cases the baby is born with a small head and a characteristic pattern of skull and facial defects. There are also often heart and circulatory disorders, abnormally small eyes and limb defects. The baby is of low birth weight, and there is intellectual retardation and learning difficulties. Pregnant women are now generally advised not to drink alcohol, especially during the early stages of their pregnancy.

foetal distress a term used to describe an infant experiencing difficulties during labour, which is marked by an abnormal heartbeat and is often caused by a lack of oxygen. It generally necessitates a speedy delivery of the infant, possibly by CAESARIAN SECTION.

foetal presentation the part of a baby that first appears in the pelvis during labour. This is normally the head, a cephalic presentation, but may be another part, i.e. BREECH. Both of these categories are further subdivided according to precisely which part appears in the pelvis.

foetus any unborn mammal but more specifically a developing human baby after the eighth week of pregnancy.

fontanelle an opening in the skull of a newborn or young infant in whom the bone is not wholly formed and the sutures are incompletely fused. The largest of these is the *anterior fontanelle*, which has an area of about 2.5 sq cm at birth. In addition, there is a small *posterior fontanelle* at the back of the baby's skull. The fontanelles gradually close as bone is formed and are completely fused by the age of 18 months. If a baby is unwell, for example with a FEVER, the fontanelle becomes tense and may even bulge. If an infant is suffering from DIARRHOEA and is possibly DEHYDRATED, the fontanelle sinks in and looks abnormally depressed.

food additives substances in the form of colourings, flavourings and preservatives that are widely used in food manufacturing.

It appears to be the case that some of these substances cause adverse reactions in children, which usually take the form of uncontrolled, wild behaviour or hyperactivity (*see* ATTENTION DEFICIT DISORDER; HYPERACTIVITY). Food colourings such as those used in drinks and sweets appear to be particularly suspect, and some manufacturers have responded by withdrawing these substances from their products. The foods in which additives are used are generally highly processed and should form only a small proportion of the overall diet. They are usually very popular and should not cause problems for the majority of children if they are only eaten as an occasional treat.

forced feeding compulsory feeding, for example by means of a naso-gastric tube, which may be used as a last resort, especially in extreme cases of ANOREXIA NERVOSA.

forceps delivery a method of delivering a baby quickly, using specially designed obstetric forceps that fit around the head. They are used when a problem has arisen during labour, such as when the baby is short of oxygen or experiencing FOETAL DISTRESS, or if there is maternal exhaustion or uterine inertia.

foreign body it is quite common for small children to swallow a small object or even to insert one into an orifice, such as the ear, in which it then becomes stuck. Inhalation and choking on a small object placed in the mouth is another risk for the very young. If a parent suspects that a child has a problem of this nature then medical attention should be sought so that the appropriate action can be taken. Even with great vigilance, it is extremely difficult always to prevent little children from picking up small objects such as beads or stones, which often seem to hold a particular fascination. Fortunately most children do not come to any harm and if a problem does arise it can usually be successfully dealt with.

fragile X syndrome *see* X-LINKED MENTAL RETARDATION.

fraternal twins *see* DIZYGOTIC TWINS.

Friedreich's ataxia an inherited disorder producing gradual degeneration (sclerosis) of the nerve cells of the spinal cord and brain. It usually appears in children aged between five and 15 and is a genetic disorder caused by a recessive gene on chromosome 9. The initial symptoms include an unsteady walk and loss of the knee-jerk reflex, followed by slurring of speech or other impairment. As the condition progresses there is tremor, severe arching of the feet and curvature of the spine. The symptoms are increasingly disabling and are frequently accompanied by progressive heart disease. There is no cure or specific treatment to halt the progression of the disease. Treatment is aimed at relieving the effects of the symptoms and endeavouring to keep the child as active as possible.

fructose-1, 6-diphosphate deficiency a rare inherited disorder in which there is a lack of the enzyme fructose-1, 6-diphosphatase. This enzyme is an essential component of a metabolic process called gluconeogenesis, which is carried out by the liver. This results in a lack of glucose in the blood and is rectified by ensuring that there is a regular dietary intake of glucose. There is a risk of hypoglycaemic coma, which is treated by giving glucose intravenously.

fructosuria a rare, benign, inherited abnormality in which there is a deficiency of the enzyme fructokinase, which breaks down fructose or fruit sugar. The result of this is that there are abnormally high levels of fructose in the child's urine and blood but no treatment is needed.

fused pelvic kidney *see* KIDNEY DEFECTS.

G

galactosaemia a group of hereditary recessive disorders resulting in faulty metabolism of galactose (an important sugar found in certain body tissues and occurring in milk and some other foods). Symptoms depend on the exact nature of the disorder but appear soon after birth once the infant is receiving milk. They include VOMITING, jaundice, enlargement of the liver and spleen, cataracts, growth retardation, fluid retention and intellectual impairment. However, these can be prevented by prompt diagnosis and treatment, particularly if the trait has been detected in the mother before or during pregnancy. It is necessary to exclude galactose completely from the diet for life, and milk substitutes must be used for early feeding.

galactose epimerase deficiency a rare inherited disorder that is similar to GALACTOSAEMIA but in a milder form may affect only red blood cells. Treatment depends on the severity but is similar to that given for galactosaemia.

galactosyl ceramide lipidosis an extremely rare and ultimately lethal inherited, CONGENITAL abnormality involving the metabolism of lipids (fats). It causes blindness, deafness, paralysis and general retardation, unfortunately with no prospect of cure.

gastroenteritis *see* ACUTE INFECTIOUS GASTROENTERITIS.

gavage feeding feeding through a nasogastric tube, which is frequently necessary for premature babies or newborn infants who are ill and require intensive care.

gender identity disorder an uncommon, psychiatric disorder in which a child is extremely uncomfortable with his or her gender. Frequently, the child is convinced that he or she has been born into the wrong body and more correctly belongs to the opposite sex. The child usually rejects everything associated with his or her biological sex, and this becomes apparent in the choice of clothes, games, toys and friends. In both boys and girls, gender identify disorder usually appears in early childhood about the age of three to four. The majority of affected children become more comfortable with their biological gender once they reach puberty. However, a few retain their feeling of 'wrongness' and eventually seek treatment and surgery to change their sex. Treatment in childhood is by means of psychotherapy to try to help the child to accept his or her biological gender.

genu varum *see* BOW LEGS.

genu valgum *see* KNOCK KNEES.

German measles *or* **rubella** a highly infectious viral disease, occurring mainly in childhood, which is very mild in its effect and involves the skin, respiratory system and lymph glands in the neck. There is an incubation period of two or three weeks before symptoms appear, which include headache, shivering, sore throat and slight FEVER. There is some swelling of the glands in the neck, and soon afterwards a rash of tiny pink spots appears, initially on the face and/or neck but subsequently spreading over the body. The rash disappears after about one week, but the child remains infectious for three or four more days. The symptoms are usually mild and may pass unnoticed, and it may be difficult to diagnose the disease in the early stages. The most marked feature, albeit short-lived, is the swelling of the neck.

No specific treatment is needed other than keeping the child at home until three or four days after the spots have disappeared to limit the spread of the infection. Mild painkillers and bed rest are usually all that is required to relieve discomfort. The child should be encouraged to drink plenty of fluids and eat a normal diet. Recovery is normally complete within one week or ten days.

An attack of the infection normally confers lifelong immunity. However, German measles poses a risk to a developing FOETUS in the early stages of pregnancy if the mother catches the infection. Abnormalities that can arise include cardiac defects, DEAFNESS, mental impairment and cataracts. In order to limit these risks, all young girls in the UK are offered routine immunisation around the age of 12 or 13. A woman who is considering pregnancy and who is unsure of her status with regard to German measles can have a simple blood test to establish whether she is immune or not and be vaccinated if necessary.

gestational age the age of a FOETUS or newborn baby counted in weeks, in which the fixed reference point is the first day of the last menstrual period of the mother. A newborn baby may be either small for its gestational age (SGA) or large for its gestational age (LGA), and both these conditions can cause problems.

The SGA infant has usually been subjected to conditions that have retarded its growth in the womb, generally after the 32nd week of gestation. These conditions include disorders of the placenta, which may be caused by maternal disease, infections such as RUBELLA, and CYTOMEGALOVIRUS, or parasitic infestation with *Toxoplasma gondii* (*see* CONGENITAL TOXOPLASMOSIS). Maternal abuse of DRUGS and ALCOHOL and SMOKING are other reasons why a baby may be SGA. Infants who are SGA through placental insufficiency run an increased risk of oxygen deprivation and ASPHYXIA before and immediately after birth. There is also an increased risk of MECONIUM ASPIRATION SYNDROME. Since such a baby is completely mature, the outlook is usually quite good as long as these problems can be effectively treated (*compare* PREMATURE BABY). However, if SGA has arisen for some other reason, the child may continue to be affected in some way. Immediately after birth, SGA infants require special care and monitoring and are particularly likely to develop HYPOGLYCAEMIA.

The most common reason for an infant being LGA is maternal DIABETES MELLITUS, especially if this has not been strictly controlled. Such a baby is usually overweight and often responds poorly, is difficult to feed and is prone to the development of HYPOGLYCAEMIA and HYPERBILIRUBINAEMIA. There may be problems with the lungs and an increased risk of RESPIRATORY DISTRESS SYNDROME. As with SGA, an LGA baby requires careful monitoring and special care following birth.

GH *see* GROWTH HORMONE.

Gilles de la Tourette syndrome an uncommon neurological and psychological abnormality of unknown cause that usually begins in childhood. The child develops various tics (involuntary muscular twitches) of the face and arms, and speech is also affected. The condition generally worsens to include shouting, grunting and involuntary obscene speech. Various drugs may be used in treatment, including major tranquillisers such as pimozide.

glandular fever *or* **infectious mononucleosis** an infectious viral disease that can run quite a prolonged course and is fairly common in adolescent children and young adults. The disease is caused by the Epstein-Barr virus, which is contracted from close physical contact (e.g. kissing) with an infected person. It is thought to be more prevalent in young people through the nature of its transmission and because, in adolescence, the immune system is not completely mature. The virus affects the liver, spleen, lymph nodes and throat, and has an incubation period of about one week. Symptoms include a sore throat, swelling of lymph nodes in the neck, armpits and groin, FEVER, headache, loss of appetite and fatigue. The liver and spleen may become enlarged, and occasionally JAUNDICE develops. The child feels generally unwell and tired, and diagnosis is made by a blood test that reveals abnormally high numbers of monocytes (white blood cells).

Treatment consists of bed rest and painkillers to relieve symptoms, as advised by a doctor. The child should be encouraged to drink plenty of fluids and eat a good, balanced diet. Recovery may take many weeks and the sufferer may continue to feel unusually tired for some considerable time. Complications are rare but exceptionally include a ruptured spleen, which is an emergency requiring surgery and hospitalisation.

glomerulonephritis (kidney inflammation), acute, post-infectious *and* **chronic glomerulonephritis** inflammation of the glomeruli of the kidneys. A glomerulus is a small, round knot of blood capillaries that brings water, salts, urea and other waste products to the kidney tubules so that this material can be filtered and excreted. Each kidney contains about 1,000,000 glomeruli. Glomerulonephritis is most common in children aged from 1 to 11 years. The cause of acute or post-infectious glomerulonephritis is the deposition of soluble immune complexes in the walls of the fine capillary blood vessels of the glomeruli. These are formed as a result of the activation of the body's immune system by ANTI-GENS (substances foreign to the body). The antigens responsible are usually streptococcal bacteria, which have already caused a sore throat. The child usually develops glomerulonephritis two or three weeks after an initial streptococcal throat infection. Hence, there is a potential risk of this condition following as a complication of respiratory infections known to involve streptococcus bacteria.

Symptoms include oedema (fluid retention) with swelling of the eyelids, face and ankles, raised blood pressure and a reduction in the amount of urine passed, which contains protein, blood and albumin. The child is likely to feel generally restless and unwell, may be feverish and have pains and headaches and suffer from VOMITING, nausea and loss of appetite. Treatment is aimed at maintaining the salt/water balance of the body. While the kidneys are producing small amounts of urine, fluid and salt intake need to be restricted. The amount of fluids drunk can be gradually increased as the kidneys recover and the output of urine becomes greater. The child must be kept in bed as this maintains a good supply of blood to the kidneys. Penicillin or another antibiotic is usually given to kill off the bacteria responsible for the initial infection. Recovery is normally complete but may take several weeks.Chronic glomerulonephritis is a very serious condition resulting from other causes and produces symptoms of renal failure. There is nausea and vomiting, pains in muscles and bones, fatigue and the production of large amounts of urine. Treatment is by means of kidney dialysis and hospital care. A kidney transplant operation may eventually be needed.

glue ear *or* **secretory otitis media** an accumulation of a persistent, sticky fluid in the middle ear, along with inflammation, resulting from recurrent middle ear infections. This condition is very common in young children and can be a cause of DEAFNESS, hindering the child's development and progress in school. It is often associated with enlarged adenoids and produces symptoms of pain, feelings of heaviness in the head, FEVER and malaise. Treatment is by means of antibiotics to clear up the causal bacterial infection, but the condition tends to be persistent. In severe cases, surgery may be needed to insert a grommet. This is a small tube with a lip at either end which is inserted through the eardrum to permit the drainage of fluid from the middle ear. The adenoids may need to be removed as well. Glue ear is much more common in children whose parents are smokers. Passive inhalation of smoke lowers a child's resistance to respiratory complaints from which ear infections may arise.

gluten enteropathy *see* COELIAC DISEASE.

glycogen storage diseases any one of several rare, recessive, inherited disorders in which one or more of the enzymes involved in the processing of glycogen are absent. Glycogen, which is sometimes called animal starch, is an extremely important substance in the body, acting as a source of stored energy, mainly in the liver. Glycogen storage diseases vary in severity and the age at which symptoms start to become apparent. Symptoms also vary depending on the type of disease present. Symptoms include enlargement of the liver, but many other tissues and organs may be affected, especially the kidneys, heart, muscles and blood. There may be severe hypoglycaemia (a lack of glucose in the blood), retardation of growth and other metabolic disturbances. JAUNDICE and muscular cramps may arise and also infections of the digestive system. Treatment consists of careful attention to the diet and special feeding, although this is not effective in all cases.

gonorrhoeal conjunctivitis a serious form of conjunctivitis caused by the bacteria responsible for gonorrhoea. It may be contracted by a baby as it passes through the birth canal if the mother has gonorrhoea. This used to be a significant cause of blindness in infancy but has now been largely eradicated by modern antibiotic treatment.

grand mal *see* EPILEPSY.

grasp reflex a reflex present in newborn and very young babies in which the child's fingers curl round and hold an object such as a finger which is presented to them.

graze *see* ABRASION.

greenstick fracture a type of fracture that may occur in a child in whom the bones are still soft and flexible. The bone is not broken completely because it is able to bend. The break affects the outer arc of the bend and a greenstick fracture usually heals quite quickly and effectively.

Grönblad-Strandberg syndrome see PSEUDOXANTHOMA ELASTICUM.

growing pains rheumatic-like pains that may occur in the joints and muscles of children and have traditionally been attributed to phases of rapid growth. They are usually not serious, although they can be troublesome and may have a number of different causes, including fatigue, bad posture and STRESS. They should always be the subject of medical investigation to rule out the possibility of a more serious disorder such as a bone disease, which has not hitherto been diagnosed.

growth hormone, somatotrophin *or* **GH** a hormone produced by the anterior pituitary gland at the base of the brain, which controls protein synthesis in muscles and hence increase in mass, and the growth of the long bones in the arms and legs. Low levels of GH may result in DWARFISM in children while excess production can produce gigantism or acromegaly.

Guthrie test a test carried out on a small blood sample obtained from a newborn baby in order to detect PHENYLKETONURIA.

H

habitual hyperthermia a persistent disorder that occasionally arises in girls in which there is FEVER, aches and pains, digestive upset and headaches. The cause is not known.

haemoglobinopathy any one of a group of inherited disorders of haemoglobin (the pigment in red blood cells which carries oxygen), the best known example of which is SICKLE CELL ANAEMIA.

haemolytic disease of the newborn a serious disease that may affect FOETUSES and newborn babies and is characterised by haemolysis (destruction of red blood cells). Symptoms include ANAEMIA, JAUNDICE and oedema (fluid retention), which is called HYDROPS FOETALIS. The levels of a pigment called bilirubin, derived from haemoglobin in red blood cells, build up in the baby's blood, and this can cause brain damage if the condition is left untreated. The most common cause is incompatibility between the blood of the mother and that of the baby, involving the RHESUS FACTOR (Rh factor). Generally, the baby has Rh-positive red blood cells (i.e. they contain the Rhesus factor) while those of the mother are Rh-negative. During the pregnancy, the mother's immune system produces antibodies to the Rh factor present in the foetal blood, and these are passed to the foetus in the blood circulation via the placenta. This then causes the destruction or haemolysis of the baby's red blood cells. More rarely, other blood group incompatibilities may be the cause.

High levels of bilirubin in the blood are treated by placing the baby under special lamps that deliver ultraviolet light (photo-therapy). Alternatively, in severe cases it may be necessary to change the baby's blood completely by giving an exchange blood transfusion. In this case, the whole of the baby's blood is replaced with Rh-negative blood of the correct ABO blood group. The incidence of the disease has been greatly reduced by giving a Rh-negative mother an injection of a substance called anti-D immunoglobulin following the birth of a Rh-positive baby. This prevents the formation of the antibodies that may harm any subsequent baby, and it is also given to Rh-negative women following miscarriages or abortions. The Rh status of a woman is always established during, if not before, pregnancy, so that any potential problems can be identified and monitored.

haemolytic uraemic syndrome (HUS) a rare group of childhood illnesses that cause a breakdown of red blood cells and a build up of waste products in the blood. The incidence is about 1 to 1.5 in every 100,000 children, with those aged less than 5 years being at particular risk. In the worst cases, HUS can cause acute kidney failure. There are three types and the two most prevalent forms arise either after a chest infection caused by pneumococcal bacteria or following gastroenteritis caused by *Escherichia coli 0157*. This form is preceded by an acute bout of gastroenteritis in which bloody diarrhoea has been passed. It is sometimes called typical HUS or diarrhoea positive HUS.

The third, much rarer type of HUS is termed atypical and it can arise following some other kind of infection or spontaneously, for no obvious reason. In all types of HUS, red blood cells become fragmented and the number of platelets also decline as they are increasingly used up in the body's attempt to produce clotting. The child becomes pale, anaemic and tired with nosebleeds and bruising being commonly present. The small clots that are formed typically clog up blood vessels in the kidneys so that their normal filtering function is disrupted. Urine production may be completely shut down and the consequent fluid retention causes swelling and a rise in blood pressure. Hospital treatment is required with fluids and electrolytes given intravenously to combat dehydration and a blood transfusion may be needed. Intensive monitoring of the child's condition and frequent blood tests are needed. In less severe cases, the platelet level begins to rise and there is a gradual recovery. But severely affected children may need kidney dialysis and there is a risk that the small blood clots may lodge elsewhere, such as in the brain. A very small percentage of children sustain long-term kidney damage and this is especially a risk in those who have atypical HUS.

Children who have suffered from any form of this disorder must be monitored for kidney function and blood pressure for some considerable time after recovery and some may need continuing drug treatment. Atypical HUS may recur but recurrence is less likely with the other forms of the syndrome. Vigilance with regard to food hygiene and when dealing with farm animals are essential in order to prevent infection with *E.coli*. A vaccine against some strains of pneumococci is now available and children can be immunised against certain types of infection.

haemophilia an hereditary disorder of blood coagulation in which the blood clots only very slowly. There are two types of haemophilia resulting from a deficiency of either one of a pair of coagulation factors in the blood. Haemophilia A is caused by a deficiency of factor VIII and haemophilia B by a deficiency of factor IX, called Christmas factor. The severity of the disease depends on the extent of the deficiency of the particular coagulation factor. Haemophilia is a sex-linked recessive disorder that affects only males as it is carried on the X-chromosome. It is usually diagnosed at an early stage, and a child requires ongoing treatment which must continue throughout life.

Symptoms include prolonged, severe bleeding following

113

wounds or injury and haemorrhage in joints, muscles and other tissues. In severe cases, there may be spontaneous internal haemorrhaging, and even a minor cut may produce serious bleeding. Those less severely affected may only bleed significantly following a greater wound or injury.

Treatment is by means of injections or transfusions of plasma containing the missing coagulation factor. Freeze-dried preparations can be kept at home in a refrigerator for reconstitution and injected intravenously, when required. Special pre-operative treatment is needed for a haemophiliac requiring planned surgery in order to raise the levels of coagulation factor in the blood. In the past, haemophiliacs suffered great pain because of internal bleeding that caused deformity of joints and muscles. Many affected boys did not survive into adult life. The outlook is now extremely good, although, obviously, it is necessary to protect a child as far as is possible from accidental injury. With care, however, a sufferer can hope to lead a much more normal life.

As stated, haemophilia affects males, but females may be carriers. Half the daughters of a mother carrying the haemophilia gene are likely to be carriers and half her sons are likely to be haemophiliacs. The sons of a haemophiliac father and non-carrier mother will not have haemophilia but half of his daughters are likely to be carriers.

haemorrhagic disease of the newborn an uncommon condition that may affect a newborn baby, characterised by bleeding and usually caused by a lack of vitamin K.

Hallervorden-Spatz disease an uncommon, Parkinson-like condition affecting children in which there are unusual writhing movements (called ATHETOSIS), rigidity of muscles and mental deterioration.

hand, foot and mouth disease a highly contagious viral infection affecting the mucous membranes within the mouth and also the feet and hands. It usually affects infants and young children and produces blisters and ulcers within the mouth and on the toes, soles of the feet and palms of the hands. The child usually has an accompanying FEVER, sore throat and loss of appetite and feels generally unwell. The patient should be seen by a doctor and should be kept away from other children.

Treatment consists of plenty of rest, pain-relieving medication and encouraging the child to drink fluids. Sucking ice cubes, sipping iced drinks or eating ice cream helps to relieve the pain from mouth and throat ulcers as well as increasing fluid intake. Complete recovery usually occurs in about four or five days. Special care should be taken with hygiene and washing of utensils used by the child as the virus is highly contagious. The causal agent is the *Coxsackie A16* virus, and there is usually an outbreak among a number of children. The incubation period prior to the appearance of symptoms is about three to five days.

Hartnup disease a rare, inherited recessive disorder in which there is abnormal absorption and excretion of some amino acids (proteins), especially one called tryptophan. Symptoms include a skin rash, neurological symptoms, headaches, fainting, intellectual disabilities and stunted growth. Treatment is by means of a good diet supplemented with niacin (vitamin B), and symptoms generally improve as the child grows older.

hashish *see* CANNABIS; DRUG ABUSE.

hay fever an allergic reaction to pollen, e.g. that of grasses, trees and many other plants, which commonly affects children as well as people of other age groups. Symptoms include a blocked and runny nose, sneezing, watering eyes that are itchy, red and puffy. Sometimes there is wheezing and slight breathing difficulty. The child should be seen by a doctor, who may prescribe an antihistamine preparation to relieve the symptoms. The allergic reaction is caused by the release of a naturally occurring chemical substance in the body, called histamine. This is widely found throughout body tissues and is responsible for the dilation of blood vessels (small arterioles and capillaries), and the contraction of smooth muscle, including that of the bronchi of the lungs.

HBV *see* NEONATAL HEPATITIS B INFECTION.

head lice infestation of the scalp by head lice (*Pediculus humanus capitis*) is a fairly common occurrence among children, especially those in younger age groups. Head lice are minute wingless insects that transfer from one head to another by crawling. Parents can become extremely upset if it is discovered that their child has head lice, and there is a widespread belief that they are associated with a lack of hygiene. In fact, it has been proved that lice actually prefer clean heads and hair that is washed regularly. The lice are harmless and the worst that they can do is cause irritation of the scalp as a result of scratching. They can be easily eradicated by insecticidal preparations that are available at a pharmacy. All members of the family should use the special shampoo on the same day, as often more than one person is affected. Many people feel a misplaced sense of shame in admitting to the fact that a child in the family has head lice. It should be remembered, however, that any child who has had lice acquired them first from someone else, and in order to break the cycle of infestation the school should be informed. Recently, concern has been voiced about the safety of some of the preparations used to treat head lice as these contain potent insecticides. In order to know which preparation to use, it is wise to consult the pharmacist or family doctor and to use the shampoo only as directed.

hemiscrotum *see* SCROTAL DEFECTS.

hemp *see* CANNABIS; DRUG ABUSE.

Henoch-Schönlein purpura *see* SCHÖNLEIN-HENOCH PURPURA.

hepatitis B virus (HBV) *see* NEONATAL HEPATITIS B INFECTION.

hereditary fructose intolerance an uncommon, recessive genetic disorder in which there is a lack of an enzyme involved in the metabolism of fructose (fruit sugar). Fructose accumulates in the body, interfering with the metabolism of glucose and glycogen and hypoglycaemia. Other symptoms include sweating, VOMITING, pains and possibly CONVULSIONS. If left untreated there may be coma and kidney and liver damage. Symptoms usually appear in infancy, and diagnosis is made by carrying out various tests and finding fructose in urine samples. Treatment is by means of control of the diet to exclude fructose, sucrose and sorbitol. Since sugar is completely excluded, a child on this type of diet usually has perfect teeth.

hernia a hernia is a bulge in the abdomen and it occurs when there is a weak area in the muscles of the abdominal wall, thus allowing a part of the lining and sometimes a small portion of the gut to protrude. A hernia may be present at birth and this is most likely to occur in those who are premature. The condition is also more likely to affect boys, with 1 in 50 developing a hernia at some stage during childhood. Hernias are categorised according to the area of the abdomen in which they occur. Examples include inguinal, umbilical and femoral hernias. In all cases, surgical repair is necessary, with the operation carried out under general anaesthetic. It is usually highly successful but 1 in 10 children can have a recurrence of the hernia on the opposite side. Premature babies are at particular risk in this respect but in all cases, recovery after surgery is normally good.

heroin an opiate drug. *See* DRUG ABUSE.

herpangina an unpleasant viral infection that usually arises suddenly and most commonly affects young children. Symptoms include FEVER, aches and pains, loss of appetite, headache, sore throat and possibly CONVULSIONS in very young children. Blisters and then ulcers usually form on the soft tissues inside the mouth and throat, which heal as recovery takes place.

Hirschsprung's disease a rare, congenital disorder of the bowel affecting about 1 in every 5,000 newborn babies and usually involving the colon. It is one of a number of gut motility disorders in which there is an absence of nerve cells known as ganglion cells in the wall of the affected portion of bowel. Ganglion cells control the rhythmical muscle contractions that normally operate to squeeze faeces through the bowel for elimination via the anus. In Hirschsprung's disease, waste passes through the gut in the normal way until it reaches the affected part where it builds up, causing blockage, pain and abdominal distension. The condition is often evident soon after birth when the baby fails to pass meconium (the blackish-green stools passed by newborn infants) and he or she may also vomit green-coloured bile. In some cases, the disorder is less severe and there may be some delay in diagnosis. Surgery is always necessary to correct this disorder and if possible, it is carried out as a 'key-hole' operation using fine instruments through a small cut in the abdomen (laparoscopy). Corrective surgery for Hirschsprung's disease is usually successful with a low risk of complications developing.

horseshoe kidney *see* KIDNEY DEFECTS.

HSV *see* NEONATAL HERPES SIMPLEX VIRUS INFECTION.

human papilloma virus (HPV) this virus is known to account for some 70 per cent of all cases of cervical cancer in women. A vaccine to protect women against HPV (and therefore cervical cancer) is being introduced in 2008. Recommendations are that girls should be given the jab in the first year of secondary school and that this should be be followed in due course by a catch-up campaign to vaccinate all girls aged 12 to16.

Hunter's syndrome a rare, inherited metabolic disorder that only affects males, involving the processing of mucopolysaccharides. It causes DWARFISM, mental retardation, distortion of facial features and curvature of the spine.

Hurler's syndrome a rare, inherited metabolic disorder that causes an accumulation of mucopolysaccharides and fats within the tissues of the body. It causes skeletal deformities, including curvature of the spine, distortion of facial features, shortened hands and fingers, eye defects and mental retardation. The liver and spleen also become enlarged.

hyaline membrane disease *see* RESPIRATORY DISTRESS SYNDROME IN THE NEWBORN.

hydatid cyst, hydatid disease *or* **echinococcosis** a cyst of the small parasitic tapeworm, *Echinococcus multilocularis* or *Echinococcus granulosus*, which can grow to a considerable size (5 to 10 cm diameter) in human organs. The primary hosts of the parasite are dogs and other wild canines, and the worm is quite common among working sheepdogs. If the eggs are accidentally ingested, the larvae hatch and burrow through the walls of the intestine, travelling in the blood circulation to lodge in organs such as the liver, lungs or brain. Small children are at particular risk of contracting the parasite, and the effects of the cysts can be devastating if they grow in the brain, possibly causing blindness and EPILEPSY. The cysts may exert considerable pressure because of their large size and disrupt the normal workings of the tissues in which they are lodged. There is a also risk that a cyst may rupture, and this can cause a severe allergic response. The only treatment possible is surgery to remove the cysts if they are in an accessible place. It is essential to protect children by worming dogs regularly and to ensure that strict standards of hygiene are maintained, i.e. washing hands and scrubbing beneath fingernails.

hydrocephalus an abnormal collection of cerebrospinal fluid within the skull, which usually arises in infancy or young childhood. The chief indication is a gradual increase in the size of the head, the growth being disproportionate to that of the rest of the body. Other symptoms are drowsiness, irritability and eventual mental subnormality. In severe cases, there may be loss of vision and hearing, paralysis and death. The condition is often CONGENITAL and is usually detected during medical and developmental checks on the child. Treatment involves surgery to redirect the fluid, but this is not always completely successful. About half of affected children survive if the progress of this condition is halted, and one third of these go on to enjoy a normal life with little or no physical or mental impairment.

Hydrocephalus results either from an excessive production of fluid or from a defect in the mechanism for its reabsorption, or from a blockage in its circulation. The cause is frequently congenital, and it often accompanies SPINA BIFIDA, an infection such as MENINGITIS or the presence of a tumour. The collection of fluid exerts pressure that can damage the brain and result in the loss of mental and physical abilities. The extent of this depends, to some extent, on the severity and the cause of the defect.

hydronephros a condition in which the kidneys are abnormally large due to having become swollen and engorged with urine. In children, the condition is often congenital and it may be diagnosed before birth or during early infancy. There are a number of different possible causes, including: a blockage in the urinary system; an abnormality of the kidney/s (called a multicystic kidney) in which the organ cannot function as it is made up of a collection of cysts; VESICO-URETERAL REFLUX (VUR), in which the valves between the kidneys and the ureters (the pair of tubes that lead from each kidney to the bladder) do not work properly, thus allowing a backflow of urine; abnormal duplication of the ureters with two leading from each kidney to the bladder instead of the normal one causing a blockage called a ureterocele. About 1 child in every 600 has both kidneys affected by hydronephros but it is twice as common for just a single kidney to be involved.

Treatment involves close monitoring of kidney function but ultimately depends upon the underlying cause of the condition. Surgery, (known as *pyeloplasty*) may be used to correct a blockage or, in the case of a muticystic kidney, the diseased organ may be removed. Antibiotics and other medications may be required in severe cases of hydronephros. If both kidneys become significantly damaged, there may be a need for dialysis and possibly, a transplant operation.

hydrophthalmos *see* CONGENITAL GLAUCOMA.

hydrops foetalis a condition in which there is an excessive accumulation of fluid (oedema) in the body cavities of a FOETUS or newborn baby. The fluid is especially concentrated in the pleural, peritoneal and pericardial spaces, hence severely affecting the lungs, digestive organs and heart. It is usually caused by HAEMOLYTIC DISEASE OF THE NEWBORN or ERYTHROBLASTOSIS FOETALIS. Less common causes include severe heart, lung or kidney abnormalities that have arisen during development. The foetus can sometimes be treated while still in the womb, depending on the cause of the condition.

hyperactivity a term used to describe the behaviour of a child who is exceedingly active and who generally exhibits wild, disruptive behaviour, is difficult to control, has poor concentration and requires little sleep. Medical opinion remains divided about the nature and causes of hyperactivity in children. In some children, however, there appears to be a definite link between hyperactivity and additives and colourings used in food, and the behaviour of those affected has markedly improved once adjustments to the diet have been made. Other children have been helped by treatment with certain drugs, although the use of these tends to be somewhat controversial. Having a hyperactive child is exhausting and extremely disruptive of family life, and parents may feel an unnecessary sense of guilt if they are unable to cope. Professional help should always be sought, and it is advisable to look for this earlier rather than later in the hope that solutions can be found. (*See* ATTENTION DEFICIT DISORDER.)

hyperbilirubinaemia of the newborn an excess of the bile pigment bilirubin in the blood of a newborn infant, leading to the development of JAUNDICE. It is usually caused by immaturity of the mechanisms that deal with bilirubin and resolves within about one week and may necessitate treatment under ultraviolet lamps (*see* NEONATAL JAUNDICE). In other cases there may be an underlying cause, frequently an enzyme deficiency, that requires investigation and treatment. Treatment methods include phototherapy, exchange blood transfusion and frequent feeding to minimise the build-up of bilirubin in the blood (*see also* KERNICTERUS).

hyperchylomicronaemia a rare, inherited disorder of fat metabolism in which an essential enzyme is absent. The result is that fat builds up in the blood and is also deposited within the skin. Other symptoms are pain in the abdomen and enlargement of the liver.

hyperglycaemia in the newborn an abnormally high level of glucose in the blood of a newborn baby. It may arise in premature or low birth weight babies that are being given glucose by intravenous infusion or in infants who are suffering from infections. It is treated by careful monitoring and adjustments of blood glucose levels.

hyperkinetic syndrome a form of hyperactive disorder of children, usually associated with those suffering from brain damage, intellectual impairment and learning difficulties. Treatment may involve drugs, psychotherapy and special schooling.

hypernatraemia in the newborn an abnormally high level of sodium in the blood of a newborn baby. This condition can arise in very premature or low birth weight babies as a result of the loss of water through the skin by evaporation. It may even arise as a result of blood or plasma transfusions or through the use of solutions to wash out catheters. There is a risk of the development of CONVULSIONS, brain haemorrhage and neurological impairment, so all very small infants in need of special care are carefully monitored for blood sodium levels.

hyperthyroidism *or* **neonatal Grave's disease** excessively high activity of the thyroid gland in a FOETUS or in a newborn infant. It is a severe condition that may cause foetal death or stillbirth, or the premature birth or death of a newborn baby. The risk arises if the mother has Grave's disease for which she is receiving treatment or if she has been treated for it in the past. Excessive stimulation of the infant's thyroid gland causes feeding problems, DIARRHOEA and VOMITING, which may result in severe disruption of the fluid/electrolyte balance and serious heart and respiratory problems. Treatment is by means of propythlouracil and possibly iodine to combat the hyperthyroidism and sometimes exchange blood transfusion. Infants with heart problems require additional drug therapy. In all cases, a pregnant woman receiving treatment for a thyroid disorder must receive special care and monitoring.

hypocalcaemia in the newborn an abnormally low level of blood calcium in a newborn baby. The condition is quite common in premature infants, those receiving special intensive care, small for GESTATIONAL AGE babies and those born to mothers with DIABETES. Newborn babies who have suffered from oxygen shortage during birth are also at risk. Hypocalcaemia may not produce symptoms unless severe and may resolve naturally without treatment. Symptoms that can arise include poor muscle tone and lack of interest in feeding, irritability and CONVULSIONS. If the condition is marked, treatment is by means of intravenous infusion with calcium solution, and later calcium may be added to feeds if necessary.

hypoglycaemia in the newborn an abnormally low level of glucose in the blood of a newborn baby. Babies most at risk are those who are premature and of low birth weight or small for GESTATIONAL AGE, those born to mothers with DIABETES, those who have suffered from oxygen shortage during or after birth and those with BECKWITH'S SYNDROME or certain forms of haemolytic disease. Symptoms include listlessness, irritability, poor feeding and muscle tone, abnormal breathing and CONVULSIONS. (These symptoms may also occur in HYPOCALCAEMIA and in infants experiencing drug withdrawal through maternal addiction.) Treatment depends on the severity and underlying cause of the condition and may include frequent feeds and intravenous infusion with glucose along with careful monitoring of the blood.

hypogonadism abnormally low levels of activity in the gonads or sex organs, i.e. the female ovaries and the male testes. This may arise for a number of different reasons and may cause a loss of function within the organs themselves and lack of development of SECONDARY SEXUAL CHARACTERISTICS at PUBERTY.

hypophosphataemic rickets a rare, inherited abnormality causing poor absorption of phosphate and calcium. This leads to growth retardation, distortion and deformities of the skeleton and pain, and requires special treatment to increase the availability of these minerals within the body.

hyposoadias a congenital abnormality of the penis which affects about 1 in every 300 newborn baby boys and is a combination of three problems:

(1) The opening (meatus) through which urine passes is not located at the tip of the penis but displaced. Sometimes, it is only slightly out of place but it can be some distance away, such as behind the scrotum.

(2) The foreskin is all abnormally sited at the back of the penis with none at the front.

(3) The penis is abnormally bent.

Diagnosis is usually made at an early stage and surgical correction is generally carried out at some stage between the ages of 6 months to 1 year. (*See also* EPISPADIAS.)

hypothermia in the newborn an abnormal, sustained lowering of the body temperature in a newborn infant. Newborn and young babies are particularly susceptible to the development of hypothermia, which can arise rapidly in cool surroundings. A lowering of the body temperature can have serious consequences, leading to HYPOGLYCAEMIA, severe metabolic disturbance and death. Thus it is essential for a baby to be kept warmly covered in heated surroundings although he or she should not be over-wrapped.

hypothyroidism – childhood onset an abnormally low level of thyroid gland activity in a young child. This condition differs from hypothyroidism in adults and may produce considerable consequences. Symptoms include mental retardation, lack of normal growth and delay in the eruption of teeth. It is treated by giving thyroxine (thyroid hormone). If hypothyroidism occurs in an older child, there may be PRECOCIOUS PUBERTY but without a phase of rapid skeletal growth (*see also* CONGENITAL HYPOTHYROIDISM).

hysteria a type of neurosis that is difficult to define and in which a range of symptoms may occur. Mass hysteria affects a group, especially those gathered together under conditions of emotional excitement, and children and young people may be particularly susceptible. Symptoms include giddiness, VOMITING and fainting, which affect a large number of people within the group. Recovery normally occurs when those affected are taken out of the group into calmer surroundings.

I

icthyosis an abnormal skin condition that is generally hereditary and present at birth. The skin is dry and looks cracked, producing a resemblance to fish scales. There are various types of icthyosis, and the appearance of the skin varies according to the severity of the condition and the parts affected. In its most severe form, an infant may be born dead with thickened, hard, unyielding skin. More commonly, the skin lacks oil and looks rough and dry, with dirt collecting easily in the cracks. The scales may be quite thin or thicker, depending on the type of icthyosis. The skin may improve in summer and become harder in winter.

A child with this condition requires ongoing treatment – most importantly, the application of emollient preparations. Petroleum-based mineral oils are particularly useful, replacing the natural ones that are deficient. Special bath preparations and creams and ointments containing vitamin A and retinoic acid may be prescribed. Synthetic tretrinoin (vitamin A) preparations taken by mouth, such as etretinate and isotretinoin, may also be prescribed under specialist supervision. The cause is generally a defect in keratinisation, which is the natural process by which the nails, hair and outer layers of the skin become filled with keratin (a fibrous protein).

icterus neonatorum a form of JAUNDICE in a newborn baby.

IDDM (insulin-dependent diabetes mellitus) *see* DIABETES.

identical twins *see* MONOZYGOTIC TWINS.

idiopathic scoliosis an idiopathic condition or disease is one in which the cause is unknown or cannot be determined. Idiopathic scoliosis is an abnormal curvature of the spine in which it is bent laterally. The condition is more common in girls (about 60 to 80 per cent of all cases), and the age at which it is usually apparent is around 10 to 14 years. It may be noticed initially because clothing seems uneven or one shoulder may be slightly higher than the other. The child may complain of tiredness and muscular pains and eventually backache. Treatment depends on the severity of the condition and its likely progression but usually necessitates referral to an orthopaedic specialist. In severe cases, there is a risk that the rib cage may be affected, with consequences for the operation of the heart and lungs. There is also a danger that the spinal cord may be affected, causing neurological damage, especially in the lower regions of the body.

imperforate anus a CONGENITAL abnormality in which the opening of the anus fails to develop normally in a FOETUS. Hence the baby is born with either a partial or complete blocking of the anal opening. There are various types of the condition, depending on the exact nature of the abnormality. Treatment is by means of surgical correction to restore the anal opening. In some cases this is a minor, simple procedure, but in others it may be quite complex if the malformation is extensive.

impetigo an infectious bacterial skin disease that is common among infants and children. One severe form in babies is called pemphigus neonatorum. The areas that are usually affected are the skin on the face and limbs, and the infection begins as a red patch in which pustules form and join to create crusted, yellowish sores. The contents of the sores are highly infectious and are easily spread by direct contact or via towels and linen. The scabs usually dry up, fall off and do not cause scarring. In pemphigus neonatorum, however, serious blistering of the skin occurs and prompt treatment is vital. The causal organisms are usually staphylococcus bacteria but occasionally streptococcus may be involved.

A child with any form of skin complaint should be seen by a doctor, and the condition may require specialist treatment. Antibiotics such as penicillin are prescribed to kill the bacteria, and scrupulous care must be taken with hygiene. Special solutions and lotions will probably be prescribed for treating the affected areas of skin. The condition usually responds very well to treatment, but because of its infectious nature a child may have to be kept away from others for a time. A delay in the onset of treatment allows the infection to gain a firmer hold, and it is then much more difficult to eradicate.

inactivated polio virus (IPV) *see* POLIOVIRUS VACCINE.

infant botulism an uncommon form of poisoning caused by toxins produced by bacteria called *Clostridium botulinum*, occurring in a young infant less than six months old. It produces severe symptoms of loss of muscle tone, lethargy, lack of interest in feeding and CONSTIPATION and possibly breathing problems.

infantile arteritis inflammation of the arteries in a baby or young child.

infantile cortical hyperostosis *or* **Caffey's disease** an inherited disorder in which there are painful bony swellings in some parts of the body, particularly the jaw.

infantile eczema *see* ECZEMA.

infantile glaucoma *see* CONGENITAL GLAUCOMA.

infantile hemiplagia paralysis of one half of the body, which may result from trauma before or after birth, e.g. a lack of oxygen or brain haemorrhage.

infantile neuroaxonal dystrophy INAD *or* **Seitelberger's disease** an extremely rare, inherited, recessive genetic disorder affecting nerve axons (the fine 'threads' that conduct electrical messages) within the central nervous system and throughout the body. The gene involved in this degenerative, neurological disease has yet to be identified and the condition affects about 1 in every 200,000 newborn babies. It is characterised by an abnormal build up of deposits called spheroid bodies which congregate particularly in the conjunctiva of the eyes and in muscles and skin. Diagnosis is made by microscopic examination of a tissue sample from an affected area. An infant begins to show symptoms between the ages of 6 months to 2 years and there is a gradual loss of all physical and intellectual functions. Early signs are often first noted in the eyes with the development of rapid movements of the eyeball and squinting. Deterioration proceeds unremittingly, with an early death usually occurring between the ages of 5 to 10 years. Treatment is aimed at relief of symptoms and disabilities with many methods and therapies being involved to try and preserve a child's quality of life for as long as possible. Family support is also essential in helping parents to look after their severely disabled child.

infant mortality a statistical measure of infant deaths, calculated as the number of deaths of babies less than 1 year old for every 1,000 live births in any particular year. The figure is useful as a measure of environmental, social and general health within a population of a particular country.

infectious mononucleosis *see* GLANDULAR FEVER.

inherited abnormalities of pyruvate metabolism a group of metabolic disorders mainly involving a lack of certain enzymes that are involved in the processing of pyruvate. Pyruvate is a vital substance in the body, being a key intermediate in the metabolic process of glycolysis (breakdown of glucose) and in the production of ATP, the molecules that provide energy. It also forms a stage in the metabolism of fats and proteins. Defects of pyruvate metabolism can cause a number of different symptoms, depending on the particular abnormality involved, which may become apparent in infancy, childhood or later life. Symptoms include neurological and muscular disfunction, acidosis, HYPOGLYCAEMIA, mental retardation and eventual effects on the heart, liver and kidneys. Treatment is aimed at relieving symptoms as, in general, there is no specific cure. This group of defects is usually inherited from the mother rather than the father of the child.

insulin-dependent diabetes mellitus (IDDM) *see* DIABETES.

intersex states a group of conditions in which the anatomy of the external genitalia of a child does not match its chromosomal sex or that of the sex organs. Often the appearance of the external genitalia is ambiguous and fits neither the female nor the male pattern. Intersex states can arise for a variety of reasons, and it is important to establish both the cause and the true or most appropriate gender so that the correct treatment can be given.

Treatment usually involves surgery, carried out at as early a stage in life as possible. It is rare for an individual to be a true hermaphrodite, i.e. to have both ovarian and testicular tissue.

intussusception an obstruction caused by one part of the bowel slipping inside another part beneath it, much in the manner of a telescope being closed up. It is a condition that is quite common in young children, producing symptoms of severe cramping pain that comes and goes, abdominal tenderness and swelling, passage of jelly-like bloodstained mucus, CONSTIPATION and VOMITING. Intussusception is a medical emergency, and the child should be taken to hospital immediately and not given anything to eat or drink. Recovery is normally complete as long as prompt medical treatment is given, but any delay can prove dangerous or even fatal.

IPV (inactivated polio virus) *see* POLIOVIRUS VACCINE.

J

Jacobsen syndrome a rare, congenital, chromosomal disorder which arises at conception and is caused by deletion of a small part of chromosome 11 along with its corresponding genes. About 1 in every 100,000 newborn babies is affected, with girls being at greater risk. Affected children show characteristic facial features. The face is pear-shaped with the eyes positioned widely apart. The ears are set low and there is a receding, small chin, a thin top lip and drooping eyelids. Heart defects, including enlargement of the left side of the heart, bleeding disorders (especially thrombocytopenia of a particular type called PARIS-TROUSSEAU SYNDROME), PYLORIC STENOSIS, retarded growth and learning difficulties are all common accompanying features. However, the severity of these complications varies considerably. Children are given the appropriate treatment for any physical problems that they may have along with educational/learning support.

jaundice (neonatal) a condition characterised by the unusual presence of bile pigment (bilirubin) in the blood. Neonatal jaundice is quite common in newborn infants and results from the physiological immaturity of the liver, which processes the bilirubin. Severe cases are treated by exposing the infant to blue light, which converts bilirubin to biliverdin (a harmless bile pigment).

JRA *see* JUVENILE RHEUMATOID ARTHRITIS.

juvenile alveolar rhabdomyoscarcoma a rare malignant tumour of muscle that grows rapidly, usually in the region of a hand or foot, and may arise in a child or adolescent.

juvenile angiofibroma a benign tumour of the connective tissue that occupies the cavity of the nasopharynx. It almost exclusively occurs in adolescent boys and causes nose bleeds as the tumour has many thin-walled blood vessels. It may grow and invade other spaces, causing further symptoms. Treatment is by means of drugs (oestrogen or diethylstilboestrol) to reduce the size of the tumour, followed by surgical removal. If the tumour has spread, however, radiotherapy may be the preferred choice of treatment.

juvenile idiopathic arthritis (JIA) an uncommon, inflammatory disease of the joints affecting about 1 child in every 1,000 aged under 16 years. There are three main types, each of which may vary in severity but all of which involve pain, stiffness and swelling of one or more joints. Pauci-articular JIA or oligo-articular JIA is the most common, responsible for half of all cases. Usually, the affected joints are in the lower limbs and up to four may be involved. Eye inflammation is an associated problem in this form of JIA. Polyarticular JIA is the second most frequent type, responsible for 20 per cent of all cases. It is essentially the same disease as rheumatoid arthritis in adults and it affects five or more joints in any part of the body. There is inflammation, tenderness, pain and stiffness with restriction of movement and deformity. There may be active phases punctuated by interludes of remission. Systemic JIA or Still's disease is responsible for a further 10 per cent of all cases. Symptoms may occur gradually or develop rapidly and include pain and inflammation in most joints. The disease may begin in the fingers and spread to other joints in a characteristic, symmetrical fashion – to wrists, elbows, knees and ankles. A high fever, malaise, skin rash, lethargy, eye inflammation, blood changes (a marked increase in certain white blood cells), enlargement of the spleen and other glands are all recognised, accompanying problems. Also, there may be a stiff neck, muscle wastage, disrupted growth and a receding chin.

In all forms of JIA, affected children require drugs to relieve pain and inflammation and bed rest during active phases of the disease. Hospital admission for treatment may well be necessary and there is often a need for other types of help – physiotherapy, occupational therapy and educational/learning support. It is very important for the child's life to be as normal and inclusive as the condition allows. JIA is a chronic illness that may affect life and career prospects but most children adapt and cope very well, as long as they receive proper levels of help and support.

juvenile macular degeneration *or* **juvenile macular dystrophy** *or* **early-onset macular degeneration** a group of rare, inherited, genetic disorders which all cause degeneration of the macula of the eye. The macula is the area in the centre of the retina at the back of the eye where the sharpest part of an image is formed. Hence, degeneration of the light-sensitive cells within the macula leads to a loss of central vision and a decline in sharpness of the image. The most common type of juvenile macular degeneration is called Stargadt's disease, affecting about 1 in every 10,000 children. Loss of vision usually begins between the ages of 7 to 12 years, although it is sometimes delayed until adulthood. The second most common type is Best's viteliform retinal dystrophy and this normally occurs during childhood or adolescence. It can arise unequally, with only one eye being affected at first. In all forms of disorder, there is no pain and there is not a total loss of vision. Affected children may require glasses with magnifying lenses and large-print reading material. A good diet and avoiding exposure to strong sunlight have also proved to be helpful.

juvenile onset dermatomyositis (JDM) a very rare, inflammatory disorder of the skin and muscles of unknown cause, affecting about 1 in every 250,000 children. It is connected with inflammation of blood vessels and affected children may become either gradually or rapidly unwell. Symptoms include pain, weakness, irritability, tiredness, reluctance to walk and appearance of a scaly rash, especially around the eyes and on the cheeks, knuckles, knees, elbows and chest. There may be puffiness in the face and voice changes. Some children experience breathing and/or swallowing difficulties, stomach and/or chest pains. Blood tests, MRI or ultrasound scans and occasionally, muscle biopsy are methods used in diagnosis. Specialised drug regimes, combining steroids and anti-inflammatories, are used in treatment and this is usually carried out in hospital in the first instance. The child requires close monitoring for the occurrence of side effects and the treatment period usually continues for at least 2 years. A good diet and supplements of calcium and vitamin D are also essential. In some children, the joints are also affected and this requires further specialist treatment, possibly combined with physiotherapy and occupational therapy. Some children later become affected by *calcinosis* (a condition in which chalky deposits are laid down beneath the skin) but early treatment and diagnosis of JDM make this less likely to occur. The outlook for affected children is generally favourable with most making a good recovery.

juvenile onset diabetes a former name for TYPE I DIABETES.

juvenile papilloma a benign tumour of the larynx that is caused by a virus and may occur in groups in sufficient numbers to cause breathing difficulties and respiratory distress. The papillomas usually affect younger children and have a tendency to recur, although they tend to shrink and become less troublesome at PUBERTY. Treatment is by means of removal using lasers or surgery.

juvenile periodontitis inflammation of the tissues of the periodontium. These tissues are those that surround and anchor the teeth and include the ligament or membrane that attaches a tooth to the alveolar bone (its root in the jaw), the cementum (the hard layer surrounding the ligament and the root) and the gum. The inflammation usually occurs in the region of the first molar and is most prevalent in children.

juvenile rheumatoid arthritis (JRA) a disease of the joints that occurs in children under 16 years old and appears in three forms, showing close similarities to adult rheumatoid arthritis. The disease affects various joints, which show a particular pattern of inflammation known as rheumatoid erosions. This may disrupt the child's normal pattern of growth, and often the lower jaw is receded. A blood test may reveal the presence of serum rheumatoid factor antibody (RF), which is characteristic of the adult form of the disease.

About 40 per cent of affected children suffer from the form known as pauciarticlar-onset JRA, which may cause eye inflammation. A further 40 per cent present with polyarticular-onset JRA, which is essentially similar to the adult disease. There is inflammation, tenderness and pain in affected joints, with stiffness, restriction of movement and deformity. There may be active phases of the disease punctuated with interludes of remission.

The remaining 20 per cent of children suffer from the form

known as systemic-onset JRA or Still's disease. Symptoms may occur gradually or develop rapidly, and include pain and inflammation in both small and large joints. Often this begins in the fingers and then spreads to other joints in a characteristic symmetrical fashion – wrists, elbows, knees and ankles. Sometimes only one joint is involved. Accompanying the arthritis there may be FEVER, a characteristic skin rash, eye inflammation, blood changes (a marked increase in the number of certain white blood cells), an enlargement of the spleen and other glands. Also, there may be a stiff neck, muscle wastage, disrupted growth and receded chin. These symptoms may precede the arthritis in some children.

Treatment methods are similar to those in adults and include bed rest and drug therapy. Drugs used include aspirin, nonsteroidal anti-inflammatory preparations (NSAIDSs) and gold salts. The outlook is more favourable in children than in adults, and about three quarters experience a total remission of symptoms. However, some children go on to develop ANKYLOSING SPONDYLITIS.

juvenile spinal muscular atrophy a progressive degenerative disorder of nerve cells that causes wasting of muscles, usually beginning in the legs and pelvic region.

juvenile xanthogranuloma a skin disorder in which reddish-brown or yellow lesions arise, particularly on the arms or legs but sometimes in other areas, including the surface of the eye.

K

Kabuki syndrome a very rare, congenital disorder believed to be of genetic origin, which produces a characteristic facial appearance along with certain physical abnormalities. It was first recognised in Japan (where it affects 1 in every 32,000 newborn babies) but cases have now been reported from throughout the world. Affected children are often of low birth weight and have elongated eye openings, arched brows, partially turned out lower eyelids, a cleft or highly arched palate, large ear lobes and a flattened nose. They often have GLUE EAR, heart problems, SCOLIOSIS and abnormalities of the fingers. Treatment is directed at any physical problems that the condition produces, along with therapies that may be helpful.

Kala-azar a form of LEISHMANIASIS caused by a parasitic protozoan organism belonging to the group *Leishmania*. It affects children, especially in many tropical and subtropical countries of the world, and is transmitted by the bite of sandflies. It causes intermittent fever, enlargement of the glands, spleen and liver, anaemia and loss of appetite and weight. It may prove fatal if left untreated.

Kawasaki disease *or* **mucocutaneous lymph node syndrome (MLNS)** a disease affecting young children under 5 years old, first reported in Japan but now widespread in other countries. The disease usually passes through a number of stages, beginning with FEVER, tiredness, irritability and fretfulness and sometimes pains in the abdomen. A rash develops about one day later, and after several days there may be conjunctivitis (eye inflammation) and changes to mucous membranes, such as a red, strawberry tongue and dry, cracked lips. Lymph glands in the neck are enlarged. During the first week, the nails may become pale, and there is reddening and hardening of the skin on the soles of the feet and palms of the hands. The skin may peel off, with new skin underneath.

Recovery is normally good and complete within a few weeks, but there is a risk that coronary artery disease may occur as a later complication. This occurs in about 5 to 20 per cent of affected children, with a fatal outcome in 1 to 2 per cent of cases. Complications include inflammation of the coronary arteries, aneurysm, myocarditis (inflammation of heart muscle) and heart failure. Also, thrombosis, pericarditis (inflammation of the membrane called the pericardium which is a sac surrounding the heart) and heart rhythm disorders (arrhythmias). There is no specific treatment for the illness other than proprietary painkillers and soothing lotions for the skin. However, as aspirin is usually prescribed to lessen the risk of coronary artery disease, the child also requires checks on the heart and coronary arteries for some time after recovery as a precautionary measure.

kernicterus brain damage in a newborn infant or child that results from HYPERBILIRUBINAEMIA. The damage is caused when the bile pigment bilirubin becomes deposited in brain tissue. Some newborn babies are at greater risk if particular metabolic conditions exist, and all are carefully monitored and treated if hyperbilirubinaemia is diagnosed. Kernicterus may cause the death of a newborn infant or result in mental retardation, neurological impairment, CEREBRAL PALSY, hearing and eye defects.

ketosis-prone diabetes a former name for DIABETES MELLITUS.

kidney defects, congenital various developmental defects involving the kidneys may arise which can produce problems depending on the nature of the abnormality. The most common is horseshoe kidney, in which the two kidneys are joined by tissue at the lower poles. The condition may or may not require surgical treatment, depending on whether the pair of ureters (tubes leading to the bladder) that drain the kidneys become blocked as a result of their unusual position. A pancake or fused pelvic kidney is a single kidney mass that has a double blood system and a pair of ureters. Surgical intervention is more likely to be necessary in this case because of problems of obstruction. One or both kidneys may be displaced or rotated into the wrong position, or both may be on one side of the body. These conditions may or may not require corrective surgery. One kidney may be absent altogether (unilateral renal agenesis), and usually the remaining one is perfectly capable of performing all normal renal functions. Occasionally, parts of the kidney complex may be either repeated, abnormally developed or underdeveloped in some way. These conditions may require corrective surgery to restore kidney function as far as is possible.

kidney inflammation *see* GLOMERULONEPHRITIS.

Klinefelter's syndrome a chromosomal abnormality in males in which there are 47 rather than 46 chromosomes, the extra one being an X, producing a genetic make-up of XXY instead of XY. The physical manifestations include small, firm testes with little or no sperm production, enlargement of the breasts (gynaecomastia), long, thin legs, so that the individual is unusually tall, and sparse or absent facial and body hair. In the past it was thought that the syndrome inevitably resulted in mental retardation, but this is now known not to be the case. Usually boys have normal intellectual capabilities, although there may be speech and language problems that can be overcome with special help in school. The disorder is also more common than was previously thought, affecting about one in 700 males. Many are diagnosed in adult life through investigations into the cause of infertility. More rarely, more than one extra X-chromosome may be present, and up to 5 have been identified. These unusual individuals are almost invariably more severely affected, both mentally and physically.

Klumpke's palsy an unusual paralysis of the forearm caused by atrophy and degeneration of certain nerves and muscles. Present at birth, it may be caused by injury during labour.

knock knees *or* **genu valgum** an abnormal curvature of the legs such that when the knees are touching, the ankles are spaced apart. When walking, the person's knees knock together, and in severe, uncorrected cases this can cause stress on the leg joints and eventual osteoarthritis. This condition is less common in children than BOW LEGS and usually corrects itself without intervention by the age of nine years. Beyond this age, surgery may be needed to correct the deformity.

Köhler's disease inflammation (osteochondritis) of the navicular bone of the foot in children aged three to five years, causing a painful limp. It is treated by rest and strapping and special support for the foot. A plaster cast may be needed.

Koplik's spots characteristic red spots with white centres that often occur within the mouth and throat of a child with MEASLES.

Krabbe's leucodystrophy, infantile form a rare, inherited, recessive, metabolic disorder of the brain in which there is an abnormal build-up of substances known as cerebrosides in nerve tissue and especially in the white matter of the brain. Cerebrosides are naturally occurring substances that are normally broken down by an enzyme called beta-galactocerebrosidase. But the genetic defect in Krabbe's leucodystrophy results in there being a lack of this enzyme, with severe consequences for health. About 1 in every 100,000 newborn babies is affected and generally an affected infant is poorly from an early age. The child feeds poorly and fails to thrive or develop normally. There is a gradual but progressive loss of all functions and early death (between the ages of 9 months and 3 years).

kwashiorkor a type of MALNUTRITION commonly seen in African children, caused by severe protein deficiency. It arises when a child is weaned on to a diet that lacks the essential elements for healthy growth. It is often a complex disorder, compounded by multivitamin deficiencies and infections, producing a number of severe symptoms that include stunted growth, anaemia, fluid retention, DIARRHOEA, degeneration of the liver and other tissues, skin disorders and irritability. It is best treated by a programme of carefully planned feeding.

kyphosis an abnormal outward curvature of the spine, causing the back to be hunched. In children it occurs in SCHEUERMANN'S DISEASE or may be a feature of RICKETS. In rare cases, kyphosis occurs as a congenital disorder and corrective surgery may be required. Kyphosis that appears during childhood may or may not need corrective surgery, depending upon the severity of the spinal curvature and whether it is likely to worsen as the child grows. Some children need to wear a back brace or plaster cast for several years in order to correct the curve. One type of kyphosis which tends to run in families is particularly likely to affect teenage girls but usually, it is a mild form which responds to corrective exercise and no other treatment is needed. When corrective surgery is performed for kyphosis, the operation is called spinal fusion. Some of the spinal joints are packed with bone (taken from the pelvis) in order to make them knit together and so straighten the spine. However, in many childhood cases, no operation is needed but monitoring of the spine will need to be carried out from time to time. (*See also* SCOLIOSIS and SCHEURMANN'S DISEASE.)

L

lanugo a fine, downy hair that covers a FOETUS between the 5th and 8th month of development. It is lost in the 9th month and hence it is only seen on a baby that has been born prematurely.

lazy leucocyte syndrome a disorder of the immune system in children in which there is recurring inflammation of the mouth and gums with FEVER, middle-ear infection and severe depletion in the number of neutrophils (a type of white cell) in the blood.

lead poisoning *or* **plumbism** young children are at risk of lead poisoning, mainly from chewing old painted wood or drinking water that has been supplied through lead pipes. Symptoms of poisoning include severe VOMITING, a wobbling gait, alteration in behaviour and consciousness and CONVULSIONS that can lead to coma. If the poisoning is persistent but at a low level, intellectual impairment or mental retardation can result. It is essential for known sources of lead to be removed from the home and particular care is needed in old houses.

learning disability any learning difficulty affecting a child of normal intelligence as, for example, in DYSLEXIA.

Leber's congenital amaurosis a rare form of severe vision disorder, or near-blindness, in which there is a lack of pigment in the retina of the eye and the pupils fail to react normally.

Legg-Calvé-Perthes disease *or* **Perthes disease** a condition belonging to a group of disorders known as the OSTEOCHONDROSES. These affect the epiphyses, or heads of the long bones, which are separated from the main shafts of these bones in children but fuse and disappear when growth is complete. Legg-Calvé-Perthe's disease is the most common form and affects the epiphysis at the head of the femur (thigh bone) at the hip joint. There is localised death and degeneration of epiphyseal cells, leading to a gradual weakening of the hip joint. Children between the ages of five and ten years are usually affected, especially boys.

The early indications are stiffness and pain in the region of the hip joint and leg, with later development of a peculiar lop-sided gait or limp, along with wasting of the muscles of the thigh. The symptoms usually develop gradually and slowly, and treatment involves prolonged orthopaedic care. The child may need to be confined to bed for quite an extended period of time, with the use of traction, splints and plaster casts. Surgery may sometimes be required. Once the child is able to get up, leg braces or crutches are likely to be needed for quite a time. Since treatment may last for three or four years, a great deal of support is needed to help the child come to terms with a long period of immobilisation. The cause of the disease is not known, and there is a risk of degenerative osteoarthritis in the affected joint in adult life.

Leigh's disease *or* **Leigh's syndrome** a rare, inherited, metabolic disorder of the brain and central nervous system, affecting the mitochondria (the minute organelles which are often described as the 'power houses' of the body's cells). This complex disorder can be inherited in 3 different ways but in all cases, there is usually a rapid, early and progressive deterioration of brain tissue, leading to a loss of all physical and intellectual functions. Kidney, breathing and heart problems, along with seizures, are a common feature and an early death usually occurs during childhood. In extremely rare cases, the age at which symptoms first arise is delayed until the teenage years or early adulthood and then the progression and deterioration is less rapid.

Treatment is aimed at relief of the many physical problems that can occur, along with appropriate therapies that may help to enhance quality of life and a special diet, devised for the individual child.

leukaemia any one of a group of CANCERS affecting white blood cells (or lymphocytes) of which there are two main types, acute and chronic leukaemia. Both acute and chronic forms are further classified according to the type of lymphocyte that is involved. All blood cells are produced in the bone marrow and lymphocytes are the key elements of the immune system and are responsible for fighting infection and removing 'foreign' elements that do not belong to the body. Hence the bone marrow, along with the lymph system and its associated glands where lymphocytes are stored, are the main areas affected by leukaemia. Leukaemia is the most common form of childhood cancer, accounting for 30 per cent of all cases. One form predominates, with 3 out of every 4 children having the type known as acute lymphoblastic leukaemia or ALL. The second most common type, responsible for 20 per cent of all childhood cases is called acute myeloid leukaemia or AML. The third much rarer type, occurring in only 5 per cent of affected children, is called chronic myeloid leukaemia or CML.

ALL is most likely to affect children aged between 1 and 4 years and is more common among boys. The cells involved are called lymphoblasts or blast cells and they are immature, normally developing into T-lymphocytes or B-lymphocytes. If it is possible to detect which of these is involved, the leukaemia may be further designated T-cell or B-cell leukaemia. The exact cause of ALL remains unknown but various risk factors have been identified:

- Genetic defects. Various genetic anomalies have been identified in children suffering from ALL but it is likely that these are not solely responsible for the onset of the disease.
- DOWN'S SYNDROME and certain other genetic syndromes. Children with these disorders are at a 15-fold greater risk of developing ALL.
- BLOOM'S SYNDROME, FANCONI'S ANAEMIA and ATAXIA TELANGIECTASIA likewise increase the risk.
- Racial origin. Caucasian children are at higher risk than African or West Indian children.
- Infections such as influenza contracted in early childhood may be implicated.
- High exposure to radiation and certain chemicals.

However, there is no definitive evidence that living near nuclear power plants, high voltage power lines or mobile phone masts poses a risk although this is the subject of continuing investigation. Symptoms of ALL include anaemia, bruising easily, tiredness and lethargy, aches, pains and general malaise. Blood tests, lumbar puncture and chest x-ray are used to diagnose both the presence and type of leukaemia. Treatment consists of chemotherapy along with steroid drugs and the regime is individually devised for each child. Further treatments, including drugs injected directly into the spinal fluid via a

143

lumbar puncture and radiotherapy (to the brain and possibly the testicles in boys – as leukaemia cells can survive there despite chemotherapy) may also be required. Treatment can have significant side effects and children may find it difficult to cope. Hence every effort is made to lessen these and to provide specialist care and support to the patient and to his or her family at this traumatic time. Side effects include nausea and vomiting, anaemia, bruising, risk of bleeding, weight gain or loss, lack of appetite, hair loss, tiredness, irritability, anger and DEPRESSION. Some children suffer further complications but 80 per cent of children with ALL are cured, the prognosis being most favourable in those aged between 1 and 10 years. The outlook is much poorer in infants aged less than 1 year with only a 30 per cent cure rate in this age group. AML can affect children of any age but it is less likely to arise in those aged less than 2 years. It is a disease of immature white blood cells known as myeloid cells. AML is further sub-divided according to whether the cells are showing signs of differentiation (development into a particular type) and according to the extent of their maturation. The four sub-types recognised by the French-American-British or FAB classification system are designated as follows:

- MO – a form of AML with little or no evidence of myeloid differentiation.
- M1 – a form of AML without cell maturation.
- M2 – a form of AML with signs of cell maturation.
- M3 – also termed acute promyelocytic leukaemia or APL.

Risk factors for AML are similar to those of ALL with LI-FRAUMENI SYNDROME and APLASTIC ANAEMIA being possibly implicated. Symptoms, diagnostic and treatment regimes are also essentially similar to those of ALL with the same risk of side effects. Some children may receive stem cell transplants. The overall cure rate is 45 to 50 per cent with the best outcomes being achieved in those children who are able to receive a matched stem cell transplant from a close relative.

CML is a very rare disease in children. There is a 65 to 75 per cent survival rate in those children who can be given a fully matched, stem cell transplant either from a relative or a non-related donor.

LGA *see* GESTATIONAL AGE.

Li-Fraumeni syndrome (LFS) a rare, inherited syndrome affecting families in which there is a predisposition towards the development of many types of CANCER. In 75 per cent of affected families, the genetic defect is a mutation of a tumour suppressor called TP53 which is located on chromosome 17. Tumour suppressor genes help to prevent the uncontrolled division of cells – the key factor in the growth of a cancer. A child born into an identified LFS family is at high risk of cancer and requires annual check-ups and immediate investigation of any symptom that persists for more than 3 weeks. Investigations and cancer treatments should avoid radiation (x-rays, radiotherapy) whenever possible.

lockjaw *see* TETANUS.

long QT syndrome an electrical disorder of the heart involving the QT interval (the period between depolarisation and re-polarisation of the large chambers of the heart (the ventricles) with each heartbeat. In long QT syndrome, the time taken for re-polarisation is abnormally great and this can result in a dangerously rapid arrhythmia called 'torsades de pointes'. The heart ceases to pump blood and there is a rapid loss of consciousness due to the brain being starved of oxygen. In these extreme circumstances, death occurs in 1 in 3 cases and, almost always, the child or young person has previously exhibited no symptoms and has appeared to be fit and well. Long QT syndrome is caused by inheritance of one or more defective genes and it affects 1 in every 7,000 people. If symptoms do occur, they typically arise during childhood and comprise sudden fainting, often during exercise but sometimes when the child is at rest. Diagnosis is made by examination of an electrocardiogram (ECG) and drug treatment (with beta-blockers) is usually effective. However, eventually some people with this disorder may need to be fitted with a heart pacemaker or other device, in order to achieve control.

LSD *see* DRUG ABUSE.

lupus vulgaris a rare skin disorder caused by the bacterium responsible for tuberculosis, *Mycobacterium tuberculosis*. When it does arise, it usually occurs in young people under the age of 20 years, but it can be effectively prevented and treated. The incidence of tuberculosis is increasing in the UK, but all school children are protected by vaccination given at about the age of 13 to 14 years. Symptoms of lupus vulgaris are the eruption of small, yellow, transparent nodules, particularly on the skin of the face and neck but also on the mucous membranes within the mouth and nose. These gradually proliferate and are called 'apple jelly' nodules. The skin becomes ulcerated and thickened and, without treatment, can even be eaten away in places. It is treated with anti-tuberculous drugs and possibly surgical removal of the nodules.

lymphoma a CANCER of the lymphatic system (comprising lymph vessels, glands and nodes) of which there are two main types, Hodgkin's and non-Hodgkin's disease. Lymphomas account for 10 per cent of all childhood cancers with Hodgkin's disease being more prevalent among teenage children, with boys at slightly greater risk. Non-Hodgkin's is more likely to occur in young children. Both types of disease are characterised by the different types of white blood cell (lymphocyte) that are involved. In Hodgkin's lymphoma, an unusual type of cell called Reed-Sternberg is involved and is a distinguishing feature. The exact cause of lymphoma is not known but there is a genetic element and also, an association with certain viral infections, especially Epstein-Barr, HIV and AIDS. Lymphomas often cause few or no symptoms in the early stages and can spread widely throughout the lymphatic system. When symptoms do arise, they include painless enlargement of lymph nodes, anaemia, weakness, lethargy, weight loss, fever and sweating at night (especially in Hodgkin's disease). A characteristic type of fever, known as Pel-Ebstein, occurs in Hodgkin's disease. Diagnosis of the presence of lymphoma is usually initially by examination of a blood sample.

Treatment depends upon the type of lymphoma but involves chemotherapy, radiotherapy, surgery and possibly, a bone marrow transplant. Cure rates for Hodgkin's disease can be as high as 90 per cent, especially if children are diagnosed early. In Non-Hodgkin's, the cure rate is around 60 per cent and, again, the most favourable prognosis is for those children who are promptly diagnosed.

M

macrocephaly a CONGENITAL abnormal enlargement of the head when compared with the rest of the body, usually accompanied by some intellectual impairment and retardation of growth. It is caused by excessive growth of the head itself, and there is no abnormal rise in intracranial pressure (*compare* HYDROCEPHALUS).

macrogenitosomia abnormal enlargement of the external genital organs in a baby boy because of exposure to an excess of male hormones (ANDROGENS) during foetal development. In girls, this exposure causes pseudohermaphroditism (*see* INTERSEX STATES).

malnutrition a condition caused either by an unbalanced diet, e.g.

when too much of one type of food is eaten at the expense of others, or by an inadequate intake, which, in extremes, can lead to starvation. Malnutrition can also arise as a result of a digestive disorder such as a malabsorption disease or other metabolic condition in which food cannot be processed properly. Children are particularly susceptible to the effects of malnutrition, which affect normal physical and intellectual growth and development. It is undoubtedly true that in the United Kingdom many children eat a poor diet, and nutritionists are concerned about the long-term consequences of this and fear that there may be adverse health consequences in adult life.

Mantoux test a test for the presence of a measure of immunity to tuberculosis that is normally carried out on children in the UK at around 13 to 14 years of age, prior to vaccination. A small quantity of a protein called tuberculin, extracted from the tubercle bacilli (bacteria), is injected beneath the skin of the forearm. If an inflamed patch appears within 18 to 24 hours, it indicates that a measure of immunity is present and that the child has previously been exposed to tuberculosis and produced antibodies. The size of the reaction is an indication of the severity of the original tuberculosis infection, although it does not mean that the child is suffering rom the disease at that time.

marasmus a wasting condition in infants and young children in which there is severe emaciation. The child has a very low body weight (less than 75 per cent of normal), lacks subcutaneous fat beneath the skin, is dehydrated and is pale and apathetic. Various disorders and diseases can bring this about, but it is usually caused by deficient feeding. Other causes include prolonged VOMITING and DIARRHOEA, some heart, kidney and liver diseases, malabsorption and metabolic disorders, severe infections and serious parasitic infestation. Treatment of the cause accompanies the provision and gradual increase of nourishment and fluids, which is of paramount importance.

Marfan's syndrome an inherited defect of connective tissue, producing effects on the skeleton, heart and eyes. The child is abnormally tall and thin, with spindly, elongated fingers and toes (arachnodactyly), spine and chest deformities and weak ligaments. Heart defects and hernias commonly occur. They include a hole in the septum separating the atria (the upper chambers of the heart), called ATRIAL SEPTAL DEFECT, and narrowing of the aorta (the major artery arising from the heart), known as COARCTION OF THE AORTA. Eye defects include partial dislocation of the lens and short-sightedness and sometimes detachment of the retina. The cause of the syndrome remains uncertain, and there is no primary treatment available. Treatment, including surgery, to correct the associated defects, particularly those of the heart, may prove to be necessary.

marijuana *see* CANNABIS; DRUG ABUSE.

mass hysteria *see* HYSTERIA.

Meckel's diverticulum a CONGENITAL, sac-like structure protruding from the wall of the ileum (the lower part of the small intestine) which arises as a result of a failure in early embryological development. In young children, the abnormality may produce symptoms of recurrent bleeding, which is bright red because of the formation of a peptic ulcer. In older children and adults there may be symptoms of intestinal obstruction with cramping pains, VOMITING and abdominal tenderness. Acute diverticulitis may occur, producing severe pains in the region of the umbilicus, which may be mistaken for APPENDICITIS. Treatment is by means of surgery.

measles, rubeola *or* **morbilli** an extremely infectious viral disease characterised by the presence of a rash, usually occurring in epidemics in unvaccinated or non-immune children every two or three years. After an incubation period of 10 to 15 days, the initial symptoms resemble those of a cold, with coughing, sneezing, red, watery eyes and high FEVER. It is at this stage that the disease is most infectious and spreads from one child to another in airborne droplets before measles has been diagnosed. This is the main factor responsible for the epidemic nature of its spread. KOPLIK'S SPOTS may occur and a characteristic skin rash that spreads from behind the ears and across the face to other parts of the body. The small, red spots may be grouped together in patches, and the child's fever is usually at its height while these are developing. Both gradually decline, however, with no marks being left on the skin, and most children make a good recovery.

Treatment consists of bed rest while the child is feverish and unwell; pain-relieving medication and drinking plenty of fluids. If the symptoms worsen, particularly if there is a very high temperature, earache or severe headache, the doctor should be called immediately. Most children make a good recovery, but measles is not without the risk of complications, especially PNEUMONIA and middle ear infections that can result in deafness. Other potentially serious complications include encephalitis, arising in 1 in every 1,000 children who contract measles, and hepatitis. In adult life, a very rare, degenerative disorder of the brain and central nervous system called SSPE can arise and this is caused by the persistent presence of the measles virus in the central nervous system. Preventative treatment in the form of a vaccine is available, and it is normally advisable for all children to be immunised.

measles, mumps, rubella vaccine (MMR) a combined vaccine that protects children against MEASLES, MUMPS and rubella (GERMAN MEASLES) and is normally given during the second year.

meconium the first stools of a newborn baby. Dark green and slimy they consist of mucus and debris from cells that are passed during the first two days of life. The presence of meconium in the amniotic fluid indicates that the baby is suffering distress and can cause the development of MECONIUM ASPIRATION SYNDROME.

meconium aspiration syndrome the inhalation by a baby of MECO-
NIUM that has entered the amniotic fluid. A baby suffering from
foetal distress passes meconium into the amniotic sac and also
gasps and hence inhales it along with fluid. This is particularly
likely to occur in a post-term infant, i.e. one who has passed
the expected date of delivery, and the placenta may have started
to fail. Maternal pre-eclampsia or high blood pressure are other
conditions in which foetal distress and meconium aspiration syndrome may arise. The severity of the condition ranges from mild
to considerable breathing difficulties and respiratory problems.
The newly delivered baby requires the airways to be cleared using
suction apparatus followed by intensive care nursing.

meconium ileus and meconium plug syndrome blockage of the
small, or large intestine respectively of a newborn baby by a thick
plug of MECONIUM. Symptoms are VOMITING, swelling of the abdomen and failure to move the bowels in the first one to two days
after birth and pass meconium. The baby rapidly becomes dehydrated and immediate action is needed to clear the obstruction.

medullary cystic disease an inherited kidney disorder that becomes
apparent in childhood in which large quantities of urine are
passed with an abnormally high salt content.

meningitis one of the most feared of illnesses, being inflammation
of the meninges or membranes of the brain (cerebral meningitis) or spinal cord (spinal meningitis). The inflammation may
affect either or both regions. If it affects the dura mater or pa-
chymeninx membrane, which is the outer fibrous tough and in-
elastic layer surrounding the brain and spinal cord, it is known
as pachymeningitis. If it affects the inner two membranes, the
arachnoid mater and pia mater, sometimes collectively called the
pia-arachnoid or leptomeninges, it is called leptomeningitis. This
is a more common form and may be either a primary or secondary infection. Meningitis may be acute, sub-acute or chronic.
Acute meningitis, the most severe form, can prove fatal within

a short space of time (24–48 hours) and usually occurs as a result of bacterial infection. It is most commonly caused by three types of bacteria, which are responsible for about 80 per cent of all cases in the British Isles. These are meningococcus (*Neisseria meningitidis*), *Haemophilus influenzae* type B and pneumococcus (*Streptococcus pneumoniae*). Sub-acute meningitis lasts for more than two weeks and chronic meningitis for more than one month. The symptoms can be severe but develop over weeks rather than days. They usually arise as a result of an existing disease or condition, such as cancer, LEUKAEMIA or lymphoma, AIDS, TUBERCULOSIS, SYPHILIS, Hodgkin's disease, Lyme disease and fungal infections.

Meningitis may also be classified according to its causal organism, usually bacteria (bacterial), viruses (viral) but also fungi (fungal) and, rarely, other organisms, e.g. amoebae. The most usual bacteria are mentioned above, with *Haemophilus influenzae* type B being the commonest cause in newborn babies under four weeks old. Meningococcus is the usual cause in children and young adults. More rarely, other bacteria may be involved, and usually the meningitis arises as a result of a complication of neurosurgery or existing acute infectious disease.

Most cases of viral meningitis are relatively mild, but some viruses can cause severe illness, and these include poliovirus, echovirus, arbovirus and coxsackie virus. Aseptic meningitis describes all forms of the illness in which bacteria are not the cause. Usually the illness is aseptic viral meningitis, but other agents may be involved, as mentioned above. These include fungi, reactions to antibiotics or other drugs, vaccines or diagnostic dyes, or poisons such as lead. Also included in this category are the cancers referred to previously. If the cause is fungal, *Cryptococcus*, *Candida* or *Actinomyces* may be the organisms involved. Fungal meningitis can occur in those suffering from AIDS or HIV-related illness, Hodgkin's disease, lymphoblastic LEUKAEMIA and other cancers affecting the central nervous system. In all forms of meningitis there is a rise in intra-cranial pressure accompanying changes in the constituents and appearance of the liquid bathing the brain and spinal cord, i.e. the cerebrospinal fluid. Hence in suspected cases, the patients is admitted to hospital and a lumbar puncture is carried out to obtain a sample of this fluid. The causal organism, particularly if it is a bacterium, can usually be rapidly identified by this and other tests that may be carried out.

meningococcal meningitis is more likely to occur in children aged under four years, and especially at risk are babies about six months old. The second most affected group are teenagers and young adults in the age range of 15 to 20 years. Infection of an epidemic nature is especially likely where young people live in close proximity to one another, as in a boarding school or hall of residence. However, meningococcal meningitis remains uncommon, and the infection is not readily transmitted from one person to another. It is estimated that at any one time 5 to 10 per cent of the population are asymptomatic carriers of the meningococcal bacteria, *Neisseria meningitidus*. The bacteria inhabit the back of the throat and nose, but it is rare for a carrier either to become ill or to infect another person. The bacteria are spread by coughing and sneezing but are not at all hardy and survive for very little time in the air or environment. When breathed in by a non-infected person, they are usually rendered harmless by the body's immune system or that person may become a carrier. It is only rarely that the body's defences are overcome and a meningitis infection is able to develop. It is not known why some children and young people are more susceptible, but it is likely to be related to individual differences in immunity.

Meningococci cause two forms of illness, which can arise separately or together, and these are MENINGITIS and meningococcal septicaemia. Both types of illness produce a set of symptoms that may vary slightly in the timing of their appearance but are usually present and characteristic of the illness. The incubation period for meningitis is usually between two and five days but may be up to ten days. In this period, the bacteria enter the bloodstream and proliferate rapidly, releasing toxins that cause the onset of symptoms. The early signs mimic those of a cold or 'flu and include a sore throat, runny nose and fretfulness, with the child feeling generally unwell. However, the illness progresses very rapidly over the course of a few hours, and the child becomes extremely ill with VOMITING, severe headache, stiff neck, FEVER, intolerance of light (photophobia), rash (not always present) and changes in consciousness. The latter ranges from confusion and irritability to drowsiness, unconsciousness and coma. In infants and children under two years old, symptoms include fretfulness, shrill high-pitched crying, refusal of feeds, fever, vomiting and a tight or bulging fontanelle. The child's skin may be pale or develop a blotchy rash, although this is not always present. The child may become lethargic, and CONVULSIONS are quite common. HYDROCEPHALUS may eventually develop. Small children can become severely and dangerously ill within a few hours, and there should be no delay in seeking medical attention.

The symptoms of meningococcal septicaemia are caused by the bacteria multiplying at a very high rate in the bloodstream, releasing toxic substances. This causes damage, inflammation and disintegration of the walls of the blood vessels, allowing blood to escape. This is responsible for the characteristic symptom of a red, blotchy rash that can develop anywhere on the body. This may be paler at first but soon becomes red and, if pressed firmly with a glass tumbler, the rash remains the same colour and does not blanch. (This is also the case with the rash that may develop with MENINGITIS.) Additional symptoms are pains in joints, muscles, chest and abdomen, changes in levels of consciousness and possibly coma. There may be shallow, rapid breathing, cold feet and hands, vomiting and possibly diarrhoea. The damage to blood vessels can rapidly lead to a fall in blood pressure and the development of shock.

If the family doctor suspects that a child is suffering from meningitis or septicaemia, arrangements will be made for the patient to be admitted to hospital immediately. The doctor may give an antibiotic, usually penicillin, by injection. In hospital, the child will normally be kept in an isolation room, and a lumbar puncture to obtain a sample of cerebrospinal fluid will usually be carried out as soon as possible. Quite often a broad-spectrum antibiotic effective against the common meningitis bacteria is given before the test results are known. Further antibiotic treatment depends on the nature of the causal organism, but penicillin G is usually given to combat meningococcal infections. In addition, the child will receive intensive supportive therapy and nursing care, which may include fluid and electrolyte replacement and measures to control FEVER and pain. With this combination of treatment, the majority of patients start to improve gradually, with the first few hours being the most critical period. Further samples of cerebrospinal fluid are usually taken and examined regularly. Antibiotic treatment is usually continued for some time and for at least one week after symptoms have declined and the cerebrospinal fluid appears normal, with no trace of bacteria. This is to ensure that all the organisms have been eradicated and that there is no danger of the infection flaring up again.

In the case of meningitis and septicaemia, time saves life, and recovery is more likely if treatment begins early in the course of the disease. While there are some fatalities, most patients do recover, although it may take some time for them to regain full strength. Occasionally, there may be long-term brain damage, mental retardation, occurrence of fits and problems connected with the cranial nerves. Meningitis and septicaemia are notifiable diseases, and the public health authorities are informed when a case occurs. The public health doctors are responsible for deciding who should receive preventative antibiotics. Usually family members and close contacts of the patient are given antibiotics and also anyone else who may be at risk. Antibiotic use is restricted, however, as the drugs used can produce side effects and also there is a risk of the meningitis bacteria developing resistance to the antibiotics if they are widely used.

A vaccine is available to protect against meningitis caused by *Haemophilus influenzae* type B, and this is normally given to babies. A vaccine also exists for group C meningococcal infections (one strain of the bacteria), but this is not effective in the group that is most at risk, i.e. children below the age of 18 months. A great deal of research effort is being devoted to finding new and effective vaccines.

menorrhagia greater than normal blood loss at menstruation, which may also be prolonged over a longer period than is usual. This condition affects some girls when they first begin to have periods and can cause considerable distress. Quite often it is a transient phase that settles down naturally within a few months. However, medical advice and reassurance should be sought and hormonal treatment can be given if necessary to lessen the bleeding.

metaphyseal dysostosis a disorder of the skeleton that affects the growing region of the bones called the metaphysis. There is a failure in the process of mineralisation, resulting in DWARFISM.

microcephaly a CONGENITAL abnormality in which there is an unusually small head and poor development of the brain, generally accompanied by intellectual retardation.

milk teeth *see* DECIDUOUS TEETH.

MLNS *see* MUCOCUTANEOUS LYMPH NODE SYNDROME.

MMR *see* MEASLES, MUMPS, RUBELLA VACCINE.

Möbius' syndrome a rare, CONGENITAL neurological disorder in which there is facial palsy, eye dysfunction, speech problems and possibly other neurological effects.

molluscum contagiosum a chronic, viral skin disease that is more common in children and in which there is the development of small, round, white swellings. The disease can be passed from one person to another by direct contact or indirectly via towels, etc. It is less common for adults to be infected unless their immune system is depressed. The swellings can be removed surgically or by other methods such as electrocautery.

Mongolian spot a blue-black spot or birthmark that may occur on the buttocks of a newborn baby but usually disappears over time.

monorchidism a condition that may affect a male infant, in which only one testicle is present. The usual reason is that the absent testicle has failed to descend into the scrotal sac from the abdomen, a condition that is corrected by surgery (*see* CRYPTORCHIDISM).

monozygotic twins *or* **identical twins** two babies of the same sex derived from the splitting of a single fertilised egg.

morbilli *see* MEASLES.

motion sickness *or* **travel sickness** a common affliction of childhood in which there is nausea and VOMITING caused by disturbance of the balance organs in the inner ear, brought about by travelling in a car, boat or aeroplane. The symptoms are unpleasant but can be relieved by various types of medication, which must normally be given some time before the start of the journey. In many cases, motion sickness improves as a child grows older, but adults are also frequently affected.

MPS *see* MUCOPOLYSACCHARIDOSES.

mucocutaneous lymph node syndrome (MLNS) an illness that mainly arises in young children in which lymph glands become enlarged and there is reddening and inflammation of mucous membranes within the mouth (strawberry tongue). There is also an accompanying FEVER, skin rash and fluid retention. Other symptoms include joint pains, peeling of the skin on the fingers and toes, DIARRHOEA and ear infections. In severe cases, pneumonia or MENINGITIS may develop. (*See also* KAWASAKI DISEASE.)

mucopolysaccharidoses a group of genetic biochemical disorders in which there is excess excretion of mucopolysaccharides in urine and abnormal accumulation of these complex carbohydrates in tissues. The disorders are designated MPS I to MPS VII and each produces certain symptoms. These include skeletal abnormalities and facial deformity, stunted growth, intellectual retardation, clouded cornea (eyes), enlargement of liver and spleen, heart defects and lowered life expectancy. HUNTER'S SYNDROME and HURLER'S SYNDROME are MPS I and II, respectively.

mumps an infectious, inflammatory viral disease affecting the salivary glands that occurs mainly in children between the ages of 5 and 15. Symptoms arise after an incubation period of about two to three weeks. They include feverishness, headache, sore throat and VOMITING before or accompanying a swelling of the parotid gland on one side of the face. (The parotid glands are a pair of salivary glands, each situated in front of one ear and opening on the inside of the cheek near the second last molar of the upper jaw.) The swelling may be confined to one side or spread to the other side of the face and may also continue to include the submaxillary and sublingual salivary glands within the lower jaw. Generally, after a few days the swelling subsides and the child recovers but remains infectious until the glands have returned to normal. The child should be seen by a doctor and kept at home until no longer infectious. There is no specific treatment other than plenty of rest, pain relief suitable for children and drinking plenty of fluids. Acidic foods and drinks (fruit juices, etc) should be avoided and food should be soft to reduce the pain of chewing and swallowing.

Complications can arise, particularly in young people past PUBERTY and in adults. About 20 per cent of males develop inflammation of the testes (orchitis) which, in rare cases, can cause sterility. The testes may need to be supported and ice packs applied to relieve pain and occasionally, corticosteroid drugs may be prescribed by the doctor. Pancreatitis (inflammation of the pancreas) and MENINGITIS are other possible, although rare, complications of mumps. All children in the UK are routinely offered protection in the form of MMR vaccine (MEASLES, MUMPS, RUBELLA) which is normally given in the second year of life.

muscular dystrophy *see* DUCHENNE MUSCULAR DYSTROPHY.

music therapy the creating of music using a range of different instruments and the human voice as a means of helping people to communicate their innermost thoughts, fears and feelings. Music therapy can help people with a variety of different disorders, particularly children with intellectual impairment or learning difficulties, but also those with physical disabilities. For example, it can benefit children who need to improve their breathing or extend their range of movements. The sessions are conducted by a trained therapist who has a qualification in music. The approach taken depends on the nature of the patient's problems. If a child is intellectually impaired and perhaps cannot talk, the therapist builds up a relationship using instruments, vocal sounds and the shared experience of music making. With a child who is physically disabled or who has psychological or emotional problems, a different approach with more discussion may well be adopted. Most children enjoy the experience of music making and no prior knowledge or musical experience is necessary. Music therapy is usually extremely helpful and beneficial but is sadly not easy to obtain, the demand for the service being much greater than the number of trained working therapists.

mycoplasma pneumonia an infectious disease of children and young adults that produces symptoms resembling pneumonia. It is caused by a bacteria-like micro-organism called *Mycoplasma pneumoniae*. Following an incubation period of 8 to 12 days, symptoms including a FEVER, COUGH, headache and malaise appear. Treatment includes rest, pain relief, plenty of fluids and possibly antibiotics.

myelomeningocele one of a number of CONGENITAL developmental abnormalities of the central nervous system in which the neural tube fails to close. It results in a portion of spinal cord with its covering meninges (membranes) and cerebrospinal fluid protruding through a gap in the spinal column. In a meningocele, only the meninges protrude. Frequently, there is paralysis of the legs, and HYDROCEPHALUS may also occur. These are serious disorders requiring skilled surgical correction that may not always be successful. (*See* NEURAL TUBE DEFECTS; SPINA BIFIDA.)

myositis ossificans a rare genetic disorder in which muscle tissue is gradually converted into bone. It is first noticed in childhood with rigidity that begins in the spine but progresses to other parts of the body.

myotonia congenita myotonia describes any condition in which muscles do not easily relax. Myotonia congenita is a mild CONGENITAL muscle disorder characterised by muscular stiffness that is noticed in early childhood.

N

naevus *see* BIRTHMARK.

nebuliser a device for producing a fine spray, used to deliver a drug that is inhaled. It is commonly used in the treatment of ASTHMA.

necrotising enterocolitis (NEC) a severe condition that can arise in newborn babies, especially in those who are premature, in which parts of the intestine become inflamed and die. This may result in a hole (perforation) developing in the intestine allowing leakage of gut contents and the development of a life-threatening infection (peritonitis), or a narrowing (stricture) due to a build up of scar tissue. The condition can be difficult to spot but it is suspected when a baby is unwell, has an enlarged, tender abdomen and/or is reluctant to feed. NEC appears to be becoming more common but it is believed that the rise is due to increased survival among premature babies rather than a true rise in incidence.

In most cases, treatment involves resting the intestine so that it can heal itself and giving intravenous antibiotics to combat infection. This is achieved by feeding the baby intravenously (known as total parenteral nutrition or TPN) so that the gut is by-passed and enabled to rest. Preparatory to this, a nasogastric tube is passed into the stomach to remove its contents. If a perforation fails to heal or should the damaged portion of the intestine become too narrow to work properly due to scarring, surgery is required. The damaged part of the intestine is removed and the healthy ends are then re-joined. In some babies, it is first necessary to bring the healthy part of the intestine to the surface of the abdomen and create an artificial opening called a stoma. Following surgery, the infant continues to be fed by TPN until the intestine has recovered sufficiently to enable milk to be introduced to the gut, initially by means of a nasogastric tube. Eventually, normal feeding can be resumed. Infants who have not needed surgery usually make a good recovery. In those who have needed an operation, recovery time depends upon the severity of the condition, the extent of surgery and the degree of pre-maturity of the infant. In rare cases, TPN is needed for quite an extended period, possibly 1 to 2 years.

neonatal referring to the first 28 days of life of a newborn baby.

neonatal conjunctivitis, conjunctivitis neonatorum *or* **ophthalmia neonatorum** a pus-containing discharge from the eyes of a newborn baby, most commonly caused by the use of silver nitrate drops to prevent infection. However, infectious causes include *Chlamydia trachomatis*, a bacteria-like organism that is extremely common and is transmitted by sexual intercourse. Many women harbour the organism, which lives in the vagina, urinary tract

and rectum, without showing any outward symptoms. Hence
the infection tends to remain undetected and the organisms can
be passed on to a baby during labour and birth. There is an additional risk of the development of PNEUMONIA, which occurs
in about 10 per cent of infected infants. Other bacterial causes
include *Neisseria gonorrhoeae* (gonorrhoea), *Haemophilus influenzae*, *Streptococcus pneumoniae* and *Staphylococcus aureus*. NEO-
NATAL HERPES SIMPLEX VIRUS may also be responsible for neonatal conjunctivitis. Treatment depends on cause, but irritation
resulting from silver nitrate drops usually resolves itself within
48 hours. Bacterial infections are treated with appropriate antibiotics and herpes with preparations containing trifluridine and
idoxuridine.

neonatal Grave's disease *see* HYPERTHYROIDISM.

neonatal hepatitis *see* BILIARY ATRESIA.

neonatal hepatitis B infection infection with the hepatitis B virus
(HBV), usually acquired by a newborn baby as it passes through
the birth canal during labour and birth. Rarely, the virus can be
acquired after birth by contact with infected maternal secretions
or through breast-feeding. Usually the baby develops subclinical
chronic hepatitis and exhibits few signs of illness. Uncommon-
ly, an acute attack of hepatitis may arise with the development
of JAUNDICE, lack of interest in feeding, swollen abdomen and
malaise, which usually clear up with time. Rarely, a baby may
develop the most serious form, known as fulminant hepatitis,
which can prove fatal. Hepatitis B virus infection carries a risk of
serious liver disease in later life, including hepatocellular cancer
and cirrhosis. Screening and treatment of pregnant women and
vaccination of newborn babies who are at risk help to limit HBV
infection.

neonatal herpes simplex virus infection a very serious infection,
usually contracted by a baby as it passes through the birth canal
during labour and birth. Usually the mother herself has shown

no signs of a herpes infection. Herpes simplex virus 2 (HSV 2) is responsible for about 80 per cent of neonatal infections, with HSV 1 accounting for the remaining 20 per cent. Symptoms usually arise about one to two weeks after birth but can take up to four weeks to become apparent. They include skin blisters, FEVER, lethargy, poor feeding, breathing difficulties, floppiness, hepatitis and CONVULSIONS. A significant proportion have brain infection (ENCEPHALITIS) and abnormalities of blood clotting. The infection is divided into two forms, disseminated and localised, with the latter being further classified into two sub-groups, one of which is relatively less severe. However, herpes simplex infection is a serious disease with a high mortality rate, and babies who survive may suffer permanent neurological damage. Diagnosis is confirmed by various laboratory tests and culture of the virus. Treatment is with antiviral agents, such as acyclovir and vidarabine, along with supportive nursing in intensive care.

neonatal jaundice *see* JAUNDICE.

neonatal listeriosis a serious bacterial infection caused by *Listeria monocytogenes*, which can have severe consequences for a newborn infant. The infection is acquired by a FOETUS while in the womb or by the baby during, or just prior, to labour and birth. It is also possible for the infection to be acquired after birth from the neonatal ward environment, although this is not common. A pregnant mother may show no symptoms of listeria infection or she may have an influenza-like illness. (Listeria are acquired primarily from contaminated food products and many types have been implicated including paté, soft cheeses such as Brie and 'convenience' cook-chill meals.) The implications for a foetus or baby depend to a certain extent on when and how the infection is acquired. If a foetus becomes infected at an earlier stage, spontaneous abortion may occur. A baby may also be stillborn or very premature with a poor chance of survival. A baby who develops symptoms of listeriosis within a few hours or a day or two after birth is said to be suffering from *early-onset* disease. The infant is often of low birth weight with accompanying sepsis (tissue destruction caused by bacterial infection), experiences a difficult delivery and has breathing or circulatory problems. The mortality rate in this group may be as high as 50 per cent of affected infants. A baby who does not develop symptoms immediately but after the passage of a few weeks is said to be suffering from *delayed-onset* disease. A baby in this group is likely to be full-term, of normal birth weight and apparently healthy. The baby usually presents with symptoms of MENINGITIS or SEPSIS, but the chances of recovery in this group are generally more favourable. Laboratory tests establish the presence of listeria and the infection is treated by means of antibiotics, especially ampicillin, and supportive intensive care.

neonatal meningitis MENINGITIS that arises during the neonatal period, the predominant causal organisms being group B streptococcus, *Listeria monocytogenes* (LISTERIOSIS) and *Escherichia coli*. *Haemophilus influenzae* type B, *Neisseria meningitidis* and *Streptococcus pneumoniae* and others, are also responsible in some cases. The condition frequently arises as a complication of NEONATAL SEPSIS, and the symptoms may be similar or more definitive signs may be present (*see* MENINGITIS). Depending on the causal organism, the mortality rate may be as high as 30 per cent. Also, up to 50 per cent of infants who survive may suffer long-term neurological damage, such as hearing loss and intellectual impairment.

neonatal pneumonia pneumonia that develops during the first 28 days after birth and occurs in two forms, early-onset and late-onset disease. Early-onset pneumonia generally accompanies SEPSIS and occurs because the baby has inhaled infected amniotic fluid. Usually the infant is very sick at birth with a low APGAR SCORE and symptoms of respiratory distress. Labour and birth have frequently been difficult and complicated or the baby may be premature. Diagnosis and treatment are the same as for neonatal sepsis.

Late-onset pneumonia generally arises in an infant after the first week of life. It commonly occurs as a result of prolonged mechanical ventilation of a baby with lung disease being cared for in an intensive care unit. Diagnosis is made by culture of tracheal secretions and blood samples so that the causal bacterial organism can be identified and appropriate antibiotic treatment given.

neonatal sepsis invasive bacterial infection in a newborn baby occurring either as early-onset disease, within 6 to 72 hours of birth, or late-onset, arising after four days. Babies most at risk are boys, those who are of low birth weight or whose birth has been subject to complications, or if there has been maternal infection. The infection may be acquired while the baby is in the womb, as the baby passes through the birth canal during labour and birth or from some other source during early life. A number of bacteria may be responsible, as may some viruses. Symptoms may vary but include lack of interest in feeding, hypothermia or hyperthermia, breath-holding, lowered heartbeat rate, respiratory distress, DIARRHOEA and VOMITING, JAUNDICE, irritability and CONVULSIONS. Various laboratory tests are needed to confirm diagnosis and identify the pathogen so that appropriate treatment can be given. Treatment includes antibiotics and other drugs, along with intensive supportive care. Mortality can be as high as 50 per cent in early-onset disease, and sepsis is a significant cause of infant death.

neonatal wet lung syndrome *see* TRANSIENT TACHYPNEA OF THE NEWBORN.

nettle rash *see* URTICARIA.

neural tube defect any one of a number of CONGENITAL defects caused by the failure of the embryological neural tube (the structure that forms the brain and spinal cord) to close over completely during development. The best known example is SPINA BIFIDA (*see also* MYELOMENINGOCELE).

neuroblastoma a malignant tumour of young children derived from embryological cells, which usually arises in an adrenal gland and is felt as a mass in the abdomen. Less commonly, it may occur in the chest. Symptoms depend on location and on whether any secondary tumours have formed, especially in the lungs, liver, skull or other bones. Chemotherapy and radiotherapy are used in treatment, and the prospects of a cure are generally better in young children less than 2 years old.

neurofibromatosis *see* VON RECKLINGHAUSEN'S DISEASE.

neuronopathic Gaucher disease (NGD) Gaucher disease is a very rare, inherited, recessive genetic disorder existing in several different forms. Of these, types 2 and 3 are designated neuronoapathic while type 1 is non-neuronopathic. In Gaucher disease, there is a lack of an enzyme called glycocerobrosidase which normally breaks down fatty substances known as glucocerobrocides. In the absence or deficiency of the enzyme, glucocerebrosides abnormally accumulate. In NGD, the accumulation occurs in the nervous system as well as in other parts of the body (particularly the spleen, liver and possibly certain other tissues and organs). Some areas of the brain are particularly affected and they are regions that control vital body functions. The consequences are particularly severe in type 2, with type 3 being a milder form of the disease.

Affected infants appear normal at birth but serious physical problems soon arise, including loss of swallowing ability, abnormal heartbeat, muscle stiffening and rigidity and fits. In type 2, death usually occurs before the age of 3 years. Type 3 NGD often begins with enlargement of the liver and spleen, with feeding problems and failure to thrive but in this form, treatment of symptoms along with involvement of therapies and educational support can be helpful, although the long-term prognosis is poor.

Nezelhof's syndrome a serious, uncommon abnormality of the immune system affecting infants and young children. The child becomes increasingly vulnerable to recurrent infections, which may eventually prove fatal. Death is often caused by sepsis.

nocturnal enuresis *see* BED-WETTING.

non-identical twins *see* DIZYGOTIC TWINS.

Noonan's syndrome an inherited, genetic disorder affecting 1 in every 2,500 children that can cause a wide variety of physical problems and mild learning difficulties. The genes involved in Noonan's are located on chromosome 12 and in 66 per cent of affected children there is a congenital abnormality of the heart. Prominent eyes (often bright blue or green in colour), squints and short-sightedness are common features as is an abnormality of the breast bone (sternum). Boys with Noonan's frequently have undescended testicles and other characteristics include webbing of the neck, widely-spaced, downward-sloping eyes, abnormally-shaped, low-set ears, drooping eyelids and blood clotting disorders. Treatment is aimed at the complications of Noonan's, particularly at correction of heart problems, along with speech therapy, other therapies and educational support, as required.

O

obesity a child is considered to be obese if his or her weight is 20 per cent or more greater than that which is expected from normal height/weight curves. Studies have shown that people in the United Kingdom are tending to become heavier, with a significant proportion being overweight or obese. A tendency towards obesity often begins in childhood, and frequently an overweight child becomes an obese adult unless measures are taken to address the problem. Experts believe that a greater number of children are now obese because of changes that have taken place over recent years in lifestyle and diet. These include the fact that fewer children now are given the freedom to play outside unsupervised, or to walk or cycle to school. Children are more likely to be confined to the home and garden and to be less physically active than was the case in previous generations. Also, there is now an enormous variety of high-calorie convenience foods and snacks available, many of which are designed to appeal to children.

Frequently children are allowed almost unrestricted access to these foods, and this can contribute to obesity. An obese child is more likely to feel tired and disinclined to engage in physical activity and to be on the receiving end of unkind teasing at school. However, medical experts are concerned that obesity in childhood increases the risk of a number of serious illnesses in adult life that are becoming more common in younger, middle-aged people. These include heart attacks, strokes and circulatory diseases, which are all linked to an unhealthy lifestyle.

It can be difficult for parents to realise that their child may be at risk of becoming obese, but this is usually spotted at the periodic health checks that are carried out during the school years. It is generally agreed that a child should not be placed on a slimming diet but rather should be encouraged to eat tasty, nutritious meals and to substitute, for example, fruit for high-calorie convenience snacks. It is usually better to ration the convenience foods rather than deny them altogether, and to aim to alter the diet in a way that is pleasant for the child. Exercise and activity that is fun and enjoyable should be encouraged, particularly if all the family are able to join in. There should not be a heavy emphasis on weighing to check for weight loss as this may encourage a later tendency towards ANOREXIA or bulimia. In many cases, sensible changes, as outlined above, will cause the child gradually to lose the excess weight as he or she grows, and it is to be hoped this will encourage a desire for a healthy lifestyle that will continue into adult life.

obsessive compulsive disorder (OCD) a psychological/anxiety disorder in which the principle features are the need to perform repetitive rituals comprising needless behaviour (compulsions) and the occurrence of intrusive, upsetting thoughts (obsessions) which surface in the mind and cause great distress and anxiety. OCD occurs quite frequently among the general population, at an incidence rate of 1 in every 100 people, but it is often hidden out of embarrassment and shame. It is a recognised disorder among school children, especially in those aged 10 or more and it is particularly common in TOURETTE SYNDROME. There may be apparent behavioural indications that a child has OCD and in many cases, academic performance suffers as a result. It can be particularly difficult for a child to admit to having OCD and all approaches must be sensitively handled. However, referral to a psychologist or psychotherapist and subsequent cognitive behavioural therapy are usually successful in helping a child to understand, control and overcome OCD.

obstructive sleep apnoea a condition in which the upper part of the airways partially collapses during sleep due to muscle relaxation. This causes disruption of the normal pattern of breathing and a failure to obtain enough air (and hence oxygen) into the lungs. This problem is detected by the brain which responds by sending out signals to partially arouse the person so that normal breathing can be restored. The periods of arousal (of which the affected individual is usually unaware) can occur many times during a single night's sleep. The normal sleep pattern is disrupted and the person is deprived of the benefits of sleep and often feels unaccountably tired during the day. Obstructive sleep apnoea is common among children in whom the cause may be enlarged tonsils/adenoids. Certain other disorders, including SICKLE CELL DISEASE and DOWN'S SYNDROME are also associated with this condition. Parents are often alerted to the condition by hearing their child's apparent snoring and other signs of sleep deprivation include hyperactivity, behavioural changes and a decline in academic performance. The condition is diagnosed by means of a sleep study and treatment depends upon the underlying cause. A child may be given nasal prongs to use at night to aid breathing and referral to an ENT specialist may be required. Continuous positive airway pressure or CPAP is one method of treatment that may be employed. It involves the wearing of a mask at night through which a continuous supply of air is delivered from a machine and this helps to maintain the correct operation of the airways. The treatment is initiated in hospital but the machine may be supplied for home use under specialist advice. The child then requires follow-up appointments and monitoring on an outpatient basis.

oesophageal atresia (OA) *and* **tracheo-oesophageal fistula (TOF)** oesophageal atresia is a rare, congenital abnormality affecting about one in every 3,500 newborn babies in which the upper part of the oesophagus or gullet is closed. Tracheo-oesophageal fistula is an even more rare, congenital abnormality affecting about 1 baby in every 5,000 and especially those who have OA. In TOF, the base of the oesophagus is abnormally fused to the windpipe (trachea) as well as leading into the stomach in the normal way. Both disorders are usually diagnosed soon after birth and treatment is by means of surgery to correct the abnormality.

oligomeganephronia a CONGENITAL enlargement of the kidneys that is associated with serious disease and renal failure.

omphalitis inflammation and possibly infection of the umbilicus after it has been cut following birth.

omphalocoele an UMBILICAL hernia, a CONGENITAL condition in which abdominal organs protrude into the region around the base of the umbilical cord. This is the result of a failure of the abdominal wall to close properly during foetal development. The main symptom is a bulge in the region of the umbilicus, and the condition can be corrected by surgery.

opiates *see* DRUG ABUSE.

ophthalmia neonatorum *see* NEONATAL CONJUNCTIVITIS.

orchidopexy the name of the surgical operation carried out to bring an undescended testicle from the abdomen into its correct position in the scrotum. It is usually carried out at an early age, i.e. when a boy is about two to three years old, to ensure normal development. (*See* CRYPTORCHIDISM.)

Osgood-Schlatter's disease a condition belonging to a group of disorders called the OSTEOCHONDROSES. These affect the epiphyses, or heads of the long bones, which are separated from the main shaft of these bones in children and fuse and disappear when growth is complete. Osgood-Schlatter's disease affects the tibial tubercle (a bony nodule) of the knee and arises in children, especially boys, between the ages of 10 and 15. There is swelling, warmth, tenderness and pain in the knee, especially when the leg is straightened. Treatment involves resting the affected leg and avoidance of all activities, especially sports, that are likely to stress the knee. Rarely, some surgical intervention, injections of hydrocortisone into the knee or immobilising the leg in plaster may be necessary. Suitable painkillers may also be needed. The cause is believed to be excessive stress on the tibial tubercle, which may be pulled out of line because of overuse of the quadriceps muscle. This is often caused by excessive participation in vigorous sports. Sporting activities can be cautiously resumed once the knee has completely recovered.

osteochondrodysplasias a group of CONGENITAL, genetic abnormalities affecting bone and cartilage which usually cause some degree of DWARFISM. The most familiar and prevalent disorder in this group is achondroplasia. The pattern of inheritance is fairly well understood, and genetic counselling can be helpful for individuals with a family background of one of these disorders. Surgical procedures, e.g. hip replacement, may be beneficial for some children, depending on the nature of the condition.

osteochondrodystrophies *see* LETHAL SHORT-LIMBED DWARFISM.

osteochondroses a group of disorders that affect the epiphyses or heads of the long bones of children. The epiphyses are separated from the main shaft of their corresponding long bone in children, but fuse and disappear once growth is complete. The best-known examples are LEGG-CALVÉ-PERTHE'S DISEASE, OSGOOD-SCHLATTER'S DISEASE and SCHEURMANN'S DISEASE, although other rare conditions may also occur. (*See also* KÖHLER'S DISEASE.)

osteogenesis imperfecta *or* **brittle bone disease** an uncommon, hereditary disease that results in the bones being unusually fragile and brittle. There are several forms but that which affects newborn babies (osteogenesis imperfecta congenita) is the most severe. The form that is usually apparent somewhat later (osteogenesis imperfecta tarda) is generally somewhat less severe. Children of either sex may be affected, and babies born with this condition may not survive. Symptoms include fractures that occur with the slightest degree of trauma, joints that are unusually mobile, transparent teeth and bluish sclera (eyeballs that normally appear white). In addition, there may be DEAFNESS and DWARFISM as the bones are so severely affected. Symptoms range from very severe to relatively mild, and in the latter form often become apparent when the child starts to walk. The cause is an inherited abnormality of collagen, a protein widely found in large amounts in the body in connective tissue, tendons, skin, cartilage, bones and ligaments.

There is no effective curative or preventative treatment. The child requires orthopaedic support to limit the adverse effects of brittle bone disease and other measures to help make life as normal as possible.

osteomyelitis inflammation and infection of bone marrow and bones, which may be an acute or chronic condition. It can affect all age groups, but in children most commonly occurs between the ages of 5 and 14. Usually, the long bones of the arms and legs are affected in children. Symptoms include increasing pain in the affected bone, swelling, FEVER, muscle spasms, redness and warmth. The pain usually increases when the corresponding joint is moved, and the child requires immediate medical attention. Treatment may involve admittance to hospital for high doses of antibiotics, possibly given intravenously. Bed rest is needed until the infection has cleared and symptoms have subsided, along with appropriate pain-relieving drugs. The infection is usually caused by staphylococcal bacteria, which enter the bone via the bloodstream following injury or surgery or an infection elsewhere, e.g. a boil. Sometimes following an acute attack, chronic myelitis may develop with a periodic flare-up of symptoms. This may be because of bits of dead bone (called sequestra) having been left behind, perhaps after an injury, which become sites of irritation and infection.

osteopetroses a group of genetic, inherited disorders that cause an increase in the density of bones (marble bones) and defects in the modelling of the skeleton. The disorders are classified according to which defect is predominant, and while some members of the group are relatively benign, others are progressive and eventually lethal. There may be excessive growth of facial bones, causing features to be distorted and dental problems as a result of the wrong positioning of teeth. Nerves may be trapped because of overgrowth of bones. Some of these problems can be relieved by surgery but in general there is no specific treatment for the osteopetroses. An example of a fairly benign form is Albers-Schonberg disease.

osteosarcoma the commonest and most malignant form of bone tumour, which usually affects older children and young people between the ages of 10 and 20. About half the tumours occur in the femur near the knee and other likely sites are the long bones of the arms. Secondary tumours (metastases) commonly occur, especially in the lungs. The main signs are swelling and pain around the site of the tumour or, if secondary growths are present, these may cause additional symptoms. Admittance to hospital is necessary for surgery and chemotherapy. Formerly, amputation was standard treatment but newer surgical techniques often enable the tumour to be removed and the limb reconstructed. Radiotherapy may also be needed. This is a serious and life-threatening condition but new treatment approaches have improved the outlook and quality of life for sufferers.

otitis media an infection of the middle ear, which is very common in children. The child complains of earache, and in small babies this may be indicated by frequent rubbing of the affected ear. There is often accompanying feverishness and partial DEAFNESS or sometimes tinnitus (a ringing or buzzing sound in the ear with no external source). The child should be taken to the doctor, and antibiotics are prescribed to deal with the infection. A warm hotwater bottle held on the side of the head and suitable pain relief can be helpful. In exceptional cases, if the antibiotics do not give rapid relief, admittance to hospital may be needed so that a small incision can be made in the eardrum to allow pus to escape. This relieves the pressure in the ear and reduces pain. Otitis media often develops as a result of a cold or sinus infection. The infection spreads from the nasal passages via the Eustachian tubes, which connect the back of the nose to the ear. It can also follow from jumping or diving into water without holding the nose, when infection can be forced into the ear by the same route. Incomplete clearance of the infection can lead to secretory otitis media (GLUE EAR), which is a common cause of temporary deafness in children. Hence it is very important to ensure that the course of antibiotics has been completed and has killed the original infection.

otosclerosis a hereditary disorder in which abnormal bone is deposited in the middle ear, which prevents movement of the stapes (stirrup), one of the three minute bones that are located there. The stapes can no longer vibrate and transmit sound waves, which results in a loss of hearing. The condition usually occurs in young people aged 15 to 30 and is more common in females. The symptoms are a progressive loss of hearing and tinnitus (ringing in the ears). Treatment involves admittance to hospital for microsurgery to remove the stapes and to fit an artificial replacement. The loss of hearing can usually be at least partially restored by this procedure. Some patients may require a hearing aid. The cause is a genetic factor that affects about 10 per cent of white people, although not all develop hearing loss. The condition may worsen greatly during pregnancy and become apparent for the first time.

oxyuriasis *see* THREADWORMS.

P

Paris-Trousseau syndrome an extremely rare form of blood-clotting disorder (THROMBOCYTOPENIA) affecting a very small number of children worldwide.

paediatrics the branch of medicine that specialises in children. A specialist in this field is called a paediatrician.

pancake kidney *see* KIDNEY DEFECTS.

panencephalitis inflammation of the entire brain, usually as a result of a viral infection. There is progressive physical and intellectual deterioration with disturbances in movement, balance and coordination, and blindness. It may rarely occur as a complication of measles infection (measles-related sub-acute sclerosing panencephalitis or SSPE) or arise in adolescence in a child damaged by CONGENITAL GERMAN MEASLES. In this case, called progressive rubella panencephalitis, there is a gradual progression in neurological and intellectual deterioration.

paraphimosis a condition that may arise in childhood in which the foreskin of the penis cannot be returned to its normal position if it is retracted. There is pain and swelling, and usually CIRCUMCISION is performed to correct the condition.

patent ductus arteriosus an abnormal communication between the pulmonary artery and the aorta (major blood vessels of the heart). It is caused by a failure of the ductus arteriosus in the FOETUS to close over so that an abnormal opening is present at birth. The condition is relatively common in premature babies and causes a defective circulation such that the left side of the heart has to work harder and becomes enlarged. The condition is usually diagnosed around the age of six to eight weeks, and treatment depends on severity. Sometimes drugs can be used that will cause the ductus to close, or this may take place naturally. In other cases, surgery may be necessary but may not be performed until the child is about 18 months to 30 months old.

pemphigus neonatorum *see* IMPETIGO.

pentosuria an uncommon, CONGENITAL, metabolic condition in which there is an absence of an enzyme called L-xylulose dehydrogenase. This results in the excretion in urine of L-xylulose (a pentose or fruit sugar). It is a harmless condition that does not require treatment. The main problem is that DIABETES may be wrongly diagnosed.

perinatal tuberculosis a baby can acquire tuberculosis (TB) before birth via the umbilical vein or through swallowing or inhaling infected amniotic fluid, if the mother has active disease. A newborn baby may also be infected after birth through inhalation of the bacteria. The incidence of tuberculosis is currently on the increase in the United Kingdom, and it is essential that mothers and babies who may be at risk are screened and receive preventative vaccination if necessary. A newborn baby who contracts

TB can become severely ill with breathing difficulties, lethargy, poor feeding and lack of progress, enlargement of the liver and spleen and FEVER. Treatment is by means of various drugs and antibiotics, including isoniazid (INH) and rifampin.

periorbital and orbital cellulitis eye infections that are most common in children and may occur as a result of an existing sinus or other infection. These are potentially severe conditions, which can cause damage to the eye or infection of the brain. Periorbital cellulitis is the most frequent condition and is more common in children aged over five years. Orbital cellulitis is rare (10–15 per cent of cases) and is more common in the under five age group. Both conditions cause initial swelling, redness and irritation of the eyelids and usually accompanying FEVER. Some children may show evidence of an existing infection, have a runny nose or CONJUNCTIVITIS. With orbital cellulitis, there may be a rise in pressure within the orbit of the eye, which causes a decrease in blood flow in the area. There is a risk of thrombosis in the retinal vein or artery, damage to the retina itself and in the ability to see. If the infection spreads beyond the eye, an abscess or thrombosis may develop within the brain or MENINGITIS may arise. A child showing signs of eye inflammation should always be seen by a doctor. If periorbital or orbital cellulitis is diagnosed, then admittance and treatment in hospital is necessary. Surgical drainage of excess fluid may be needed, along with appropriate antibiotic treatment and possibly other measures as required.

peripheral pulmonic stenosis a CONGENITAL abnormality causing obstruction of the flow of blood through branches of the pulmonary arteries within the lungs. This produces a continual abnormal murmur and a decrease in the size of the blood vessels beyond the obstruction. The stenosis may arise as a feature of certain other conditions such as CONGENITAL GERMAN MEASLES, and treatment endeavours to preserve and maintain circulation in the branches of the pulmonary arteries.

persistent pulmonary hypertension (PPH) *or* **persistent foetal circulation** a serious, potentially fatal disorder in a newborn baby in which the blood circulation in the lungs returns to a foetal stage. As a result, there is a right to left abnormal shunting of blood and a severe lack of oxygen in the arterial circulation, which supplies all the tissues and organs. The condition most commonly arises in full-term or post-term babies or those born to mothers who have suffered pre-eclampsia, high blood pressure or placental insufficiency. A baby with this condition requires intensive care treatment, particularly positive pressure ventilation with 100 per cent oxygen and also intravenous infusion of sodium bicarbonate (alkalinisation) to dilate the small arteries of the lungs. Treatment is not successful in all cases.

Perthes disease *see* LEGG-CALVÉ-PERTHES DISEASE.

pertussis *see* WHOOPING COUGH.

pesplanus *see* FLAT FOOT.

petit mal a lesser type of epileptic seizure (*see* EPILEPSY), usually consisting of a very brief period of unconsciousness when the eyes stare blankly but posture is maintained. The episode usually lasts for a few seconds before full awareness returns. Children suffering frequent fits may have learning difficulties, but the condition may disappear in adult life.

phenylketonuria a genetic disorder that results in the deficiency of an enzyme that converts phenylalanine (an essential amino acid) to tyrosine. Children can be severely mentally retarded by an excess of phenylalanine in the blood, which causes damage to the central nervous system. A test carried out on newborn infants (the GUTHRIE TEST) detects the condition and the child's diet must be adjusted to avoid phenylalanine.

phimosis a condition in which the edge of the foreskin is narrowed and cannot be drawn back over the glans of the penis. To avoid inflammation and infection, CIRCUMCISION may be necessary.

pica an abnormal desire to eat inappropriate substances such as soap, chalk, soil, clay, etc, which may arise in childhood. It can be associated with a nutritional deficiency and is also a feature of some mental disorders.

PIE (pulmonary interstitial emphysema) *see* PULMONARY AIR BLOCK SYNDROME.

pink disease *see* ACRODYNIA.

pinworms *see* THREADWORMS.

pituitary dwarfism a condition in which a child is of unusually short stature but has a body that is correctly proportioned. There is normal intellectual development but the onset of puberty may be delayed. The condition is caused by a lowered level of function in the anterior lobe of the pituitary gland at the base of the brain. In most cases there is a deficiency in secretion of growth hormone, and treatment is by means of hormone replacement therapy. *See also* DWARFISM.

PKD *see* POLYCYSTIC KIDNEY DISEASE.

plumbism *see* LEAD POISONING.

pneumonia a severe inflammation and infection of the lungs caused by many different kinds of bacteria and sometimes viruses and fungi. The infection can occur at any age but may be particularly severe in young children. The infection results in the small air sacs of the lungs (the alveoli) becoming filled with fluid and pus. Hence they become solid and air can no longer enter, greatly reducing the capacity and operation of the lungs. Symptoms vary in intensity depending on how much of the lung is affected. They include chills and shivering, high FEVER, sweating, breathlessness, chest pain, coughing and CYANOSIS. (In cyanosis there is a blue appearance of the skin as a result of insufficient oxygen within the blood and tissues.) A sputum is produced that is often rust-coloured or it may be thicker and contain pus. Breathing is shallow, laboured and painful. If cyanosis occurs, there may be drowsiness and confusion or CONVULSIONS in children. Treatment for a child usually involves admittance to hospital for antibiotic therapy.

Antibiotics may need to be given intravenously along with fluids to avoid DEHYDRATION. Oxygen to ease breathing and analgesics to relieve pain may be needed, with tepid sponging to reduce fever. Amantadine or acyclovir may be given for viral pneumonia. Young children, particularly those with previous illness, are at greatest risk, and pneumonia can be fatal in some cases. It is usually contracted by inhalation of airborne deposits containing the causal bacteria, commonly *Streptococcus pneumoniae*, *Staphylococcus aureus*, *Chlamydia pneumoniae* or *Mycoplasma pneumoniae*.

pneumothorax, pneumomediastinum, pneumopericardium *see* PULMONARY AIR BLOCK SYNDROME.

poisoning, accidental accidental poisoning usually occurs in the home environment and the peak age at which children are most at risk is 2 to $2^1/_2$ years. At this age small children are not only mobile but highly inquisitive and still prone to investigating objects by putting them in the mouth. This is combined with having very little concept of risk or danger. Many non-food/drink items commonly present in the home can be harmful or poisonous, especially if ingested in significant quantities. Other small, hard items can all too easily pose a choking hazard. Common poisons include medicines, vitamin pills, cleaning fluids, plants, alcohol, cigarettes, paint, weed-killer, slug pellets and other garden chemicals. All of these must be kept out of reach or preferably locked securely in cupboards with tamper-proof latches. However, quite often an accident happens in circumstances that were not foreseen or while a parent was momentarily distracted.

Medical advice should be immediately sought when it is suspected that a child has swallowed something harmful. In the case of a known poison, the child should be immediately taken to hospital, along with the bottle or container holding the substance so that medical staff may obtain all the available information that will enable them to decide upon appropriate action. If the source of the poisoning is unknown, as might be the case if a child has eaten a garden plant, analysis of blood samples may be needed. Symptoms of poisoning may not arise immediately depending upon the nature of the toxin involved, but include vomiting, severe stomach and abdominal pains, nausea, headache, drowsiness, fits and coma. Treatment methods include stomach washout, administering charcoal to absorb the poison, antidotes, if applicable and other drugs to alleviate symptoms. Treatment in intensive care may be needed.

poliovirus vaccine a preparation of poliovirus given to all children in the UK to protect against polio. Trivalent live oral polio vaccine (TOPV), otherwise known as Sabin vaccine, is the form usually given unless there are particular reasons why this should not be the case. It is given by mouth in infancy and before the child starts school. Inactivated polio virus (IPV), otherwise known as Salk vaccine, is given to children with immunodeficient conditions by means of subcutaneous injection.

polycystic kidney disease (PKD) a group of abnormal disorders of the kidney characterised by the development of cysts. These are inherited disorders that may be either dominant or recessive. They may be present before or at birth or develop in childhood or adult life. The kidneys enlarge but have a reduced ability to perform their normal functions. Healthy tissue is replaced by diseased cysts, which are expanded portions of kidney tubules. These may cause low backache or sharp, stabbing pain of a colicky nature in the kidneys. There may also be blood in the urine and frequent urinary tract infections. Treatment depends on the severity of the symptoms and is aimed at maintaining kidney function and treating infections. Dialysis or a kidney transplant operation may eventually be necessary. The cause of these disorders is usually a mutant gene located on chromosome 16, and genetic counselling may help affected families.

polymyositis *or* **dermatomyositis** a disease of connective tissue with

181

inflammation and degeneration of many muscles (polymyositis) and also the skin (dermatomyositis). It leads to weakness and atrophy of muscles, especially those of the limbs, shoulders and hips. In children, it usually first appears between the ages of five and 15, and symptoms generally arise in an acute form following an infection. Symptoms include muscle weakness, especially noticed in the hip and shoulder girdles, and also in the throat, causing swallowing difficulty, regurgitation of food and voice changes. There may be a raised, dusky skin rash that is itchy and can occur on the face, neck, trunk and limbs. There may be muscle tenderness and pain, and eventually the limbs may become contracted.

Treatment is likely to involve admittance to hospital for treatment with corticosteroid drugs, especially prednisone, during the acute stages of the disease. Immunosuppressive drugs are sometimes needed and also potassium supplements and antacids. Physiotherapy is likely to be needed to combat muscle contracture. The outlook is extremely variable and difficult to predict, but tends to be more favourable in children, in whom there may be remission or cure.

Pompe's disease *see* GLYCOGEN STORAGE DISEASE.

post-infectious encephalitis *see* ENCEPHALITIS.

post-infectious glomerulonephritis a kidney infection that may occur in children who have recently had a streptococcal infection elsewhere. Symptoms include blood in urine, fluid retention and reduction in urination, and antibiotic treatment is needed.

postural drainage a method used in children with CYSTIC FIBROSIS to bring about the drainage of secretions that are clogging up the bronchi and lungs. It involves the tilting of the body with pillows or over the edge of the bed, and vigorous patting of the back to help dislodge mucus into the windpipe from where it can be coughed up.

PPH *see* PERSISTENT PULMONARY HYPERTENSION.

Prader-Willi syndrome (PWS) a rare chromosomal disorder in which the abnormality occurs on chromosome 15, affecting 1 in every 15,000 to 20,000 newborn babies. The abnormality affects the hypothalamus, the area of the brain which controls appetite. As a result, the principle feature of PWS is an uncontrolled appetite. In early infancy, PWS babies are often small with poor muscle tone and difficulties in feeding. Boys often have undescended testicles and hands and feet may appear unusually small. Later the child develops an insatiable appetite and single-minded obsession with food but tend to remain short in stature and often have poor motor skills. Learning disabilities, underdeveloped sexual organs, obesity (with its associated health conditions such as diabetes and heart disease) and behavioural problems are all commonly found. Parents and carers need to be constantly vigilant in controlling the child's food intake and this can be extremely difficult. The child may eat inappropriate substances and needs to be closely supervised. Educational support and physical therapies can help and recent research suggests that treatment with growth hormone may prove to be useful. Appropriate treatment with hormones may be needed for growth and maturation of sex organs.

precocious puberty the early development of the reproductive organs and secondary sexual characteristics in a young child. There are several varieties of this condition, some of which are associated with an identifiable cause such as the presence of a tumour or other disease. Treatment depends on cause but may involve surgery and the use of various drugs. The development of the child must be carefully monitored, but in many cases the condition can be successfully brought under control.

premature baby an infant born two or more weeks before full term who weighs less than 2.5 kg. The baby has little fat and appears thin with a disproportionately large head. The skin is shiny and almost transparent, with prominent vessels easily seen. The palms of the hands and soles of the feet lack creases, there is little or no hair and usually care is needed in a premature baby unit.

primary amenorrhoea *see* AMENORRHOEA.

pseudorubella *see* ROSEOLA INFANTUM.

pseudoxanthoma elasticum (PXE) *or* **Grönblad-Strandberg syndrome** an inherited disease of connective tissue affecting the skin, eyes and arteries. There is premature ageing and changes in the fibres of the skin and retina of the eyes with the appearance of brown streaks. The arterial walls degenerate and there is bleeding. Bleeding in the retina may lead to severe damage and loss of vision. The heart is frequently affected, with the development of angina pectoris and high blood pressure. Treatment is aimed at relieving symptoms and lessening their effects, but this is a severe condition that may cause premature death in adulthood.

puberty the period in the life of a child during which sexual maturity is gained under the influence of hormones. In girls it usually starts between the ages of 10 and 14 and lasts for about five years. There is a period of, usually quite marked, growth in height and a gain in weight, and menstruation begins. The pattern of fat distribution changes, producing the characteristic female body shape, the uterus enlarges and the genital organs develop and mature. The secondary sexual characteristics develop, with growth of underarm and pubic hair, enlargement of the breasts and sweat glands. In boys, the onset of puberty is usually between 12 and 14 years. Under the influence of the hormone testosterone secreted by the testicles, a series of gradual changes occur in a definite sequence. These are enlargement of the scrotum and testicles, elongation and enlargement of the penis, and growth of pubic hair, underarm, body and facial hair. In addition, there is considerable muscle and skeletal growth, with the boy more or less reaching his adult height by the end of puberty. A further change is the gradual enlargement of the vocal cords so that the voice 'breaks' and deepens to that of an adult. Mature sperm are produced by around the age of 14 to 16, depending on the boy's age at the start of puberty. However, maximum male fertility is attained a little later, in the late teens and twenties. For both sexes, but particularly boys, the surge in hormones may be associated with the development of ACNE.

pulmonary air block syndrome *or* **pulmonary interstitial emphysema (PIE)** (also pneumothorax, pneumomediastinum, pneumopericardium) an abnormal leakage of air from the pulmonary air spaces of the lungs in a newborn baby. It is fairly common in babies with breathing problems, especially those with MECONIUM ASPIRATION SYNDROME or RESPIRATORY DISTRESS SYNDROME, and may involve one or both lungs. It may also occur in babies receiving mechanical ventilation of the lungs.

pulmonic valve stenosis an abnormal constriction of the pulmonary valve causing obstruction of the flow of blood from the right ventricle. It may occur in a newborn baby and requires immediate emergency treatment with drugs and corrective surgery. In older children, it may be treated either by balloon valvuloplasty or surgery.

PXE *see* PSEUDOXANTHOMA ELASTICUM.

pyloric stenosis an abnormal narrowing of the outlet between the stomach and the intestine (the pylorus) due to thickening of the muscle. It usually develops around six weeks after birth and boys are more likely to be affected. There is also a tendency for the disorder to occur in families. In the early weeks of life, a baby tends to regurgitate milk after feeding but as the condition worsens, vomiting becomes forceful (projectile vomiting) and it is often yellow in colour, consisting of curdled milk that has been unable to pass beyond the stomach. The thickened muscle can often be felt and seen externally, especially during feeding. Little or no faeces are passed and without treatment, the baby starts to show signs of dehydration. The condition is corrected by means of a surgical operation called pyloromyotomy in which some of the muscle is cut through so that the opening is able to expand. Most babies make a full and complete recovery without complications.

pyrexia *see* FEVER.

R

renal osteodystrophy chronic kidney failure, causing leakage of minerals from, and abnormalities in growth of, bones.

respiratory distress syndrome in the newborn *or* **hyaline membrane disease** a condition arising particularly in PREMATURE infants born between 32–37 weeks gestation; characterised by rapid, shallow, laboured breathing. It arises because the lungs are not properly expanded and lack a substance known as surfactant, which is necessary to bring that expansion about. Intensive care treatment in a premature baby unit is required, which may include artificial ventilation.

retinoblastoma a rare malignant tumour of the retina that has a familial basis in some cases. It is usually diagnosed before the age of two years and responds well to treatment if contained within the eye and caught at an early stage. Various forms of treatment may be needed, including ongoing monitoring, and vision can usually be preserved. Those with inherited forms of the disease are at greater risk of developing secondary growths.

retinopathy in premature babies (ROP) an abnormal condition of the retina of the eyes in a premature baby that can result in blindness or eye problems in later life. The blood vessels supplying the retina continue to grow throughout the second half of pregnancy and this process is completed shortly before birth. ROP affects a premature baby when the blood vessels grow in an abnormal pattern after birth. The condition is more likely to arise in a very small infant weighing less than 1 kg and in those with a number of difficulties at birth. A baby who is at risk requires careful monitoring of the eyes after birth and appropriate treatment, including cryotherapy (the application of very cold instruments using solid carbon dioxide or liquid nitrogen). The outcome depends on severity and a few children may suffer loss of vision. Others may develop or be more susceptible to visual and retinal problems in later life.

retropharyngeal abscess a type of abscess that may develop in the retropharyngeal lymph nodes of a baby or young child as a result of an infection in the ear, nose or throat. Symptoms include painful swallowing, FEVER, swollen lymph glands in the neck and possible breathing difficulties. Treatment involves prompt admittance to hospital for surgical drainage of the abscess and antibiotic therapy, given at first intravenously and then by mouth. There is a risk of rupture of the abscess, which can cause serious complications, and so there should be no delay in seeking treatment.

Rett syndrome a rare, congenital, genetic, neurological disorder that almost always affects girls. It produces profound physical and intellectual disabilities and occurs in 1 in every 10,000 to 15,000 newborn baby girls. The faulty gene has been identified as MeCP2 and it is located on the X-chromosome. Its normal function is to prevent over-production of certain proteins in the brain. In Rett syndrome, the absence of regulation means that the protein causes irreversible damage within the central nervous system. The infant usually develops normally during the first 12 months of life but in the second year, there is a gradual regression and loss of skills such as crawling or walking, hand coordination and early speech and vocabulary. Other signs include repetitive hand movements, clumsiness and stiffness, an abnormal EEG (electroencephalogram) and EPILEPSY (in about half of all cases). The child becomes highly disabled and totally dependent throughout life.

Reye's syndrome a rare but serious disease of childhood that seems to follow on from a viral infection such as CHICKEN POX or influenza, often becoming apparent during recovery from the illness. The symptoms include nausea, VOMITING and mental disturbances that may manifest themselves in a number of ways. The child may be confused, forgetful and lethargic or excited and agitated. Eventually this may lead to unresponsiveness, coma, CONVULSIONS, fixed dilated pupils, respiratory collapse and death. In many cases, enlargement and damage to the liver occurs, and other organs such as the pancreas, kidneys, spleen, heart and lymph nodes may be affected. The child requires emergency admittance to hospital for intensive supportive care, although there is no specific drug treatment. However, assisted ventilation, intravenous fluids and various drugs may be needed to maintain the child in a stable condition. The outlook varies according to the severity of the symptoms but is more favourable in those who receive early intensive care.

The cause is unknown, but aspirin may be implicated in the development of Reye's syndrome. This drug is no longer recommended for children under the age of 12 years. The overall mortality rate is about 21 per cent, but children who lapse into the deeper stages of coma are most at risk. The outlook for those less severely affected is generally good. About 30 per cent of surviving children have some residual brain damage, especially if they lapsed into coma or suffered from fits.

Rhesus factor *or* **Rh factor** a blood antigen that is present in about 85 per cent of people, who are then termed Rh positive. The remaining 15 per cent lack the Rh factor and are called Rh negative. Problems can arise if a Rh-positive FOETUS is carried by a negative mother, and there is incompatibility between the two – Rhesus incompatibility. (*See also* HAEMOLYTIC DISEASE OF THE NEWBORN.)

rheumatic fever a severe disease, occurring mainly in children or adolescents, that is a complication of infections with group A streptococcus bacteria. It generally occurs following a streptococcal infection of the upper respiratory tract and produces a wide range of symptoms. These include FEVER, pains, loss of appetite and malaise. Usually there are symptoms of arthritis with pains that progress from joint to joint. Often the wrists, elbows, ankles and knees are involved and they become swollen, tender, hot and painful. Painless nodules may develop beneath the skin over bony protuberances such as the elbows, knees and wrists. Also, there may be chorea (involuntary jerking movements of the muscles) and the development of a characteristic, transient rash called erythema marginatum.

A serious set of symptoms that often accompanies rheumatic fever is inflammation of the heart (carditis), which can include the muscles, valves and membranes. The condition may cause rheumatic heart disease in which there is scarring and inflammation of heart structures. In later adult life, there may be a need for surgery to replace damaged heart valves. Treatment depends on symptoms, but rest in bed is needed until the attack subsides. Antibiotics such as penicillin are usually prescribed to kill the causal bacteria, and for arthritis, analgesics, non-steroidal anti-inflammatory drugs or corticosteroids may be needed. Following recovery, low doses of antibiotics may continue to be prescribed to prevent any further streptococcal infections.

Rh factor *see* RHESUS FACTOR.

rickets a disease affecting children caused by a deficiency of vitamin D. Vitamin D can be manufactured in the skin in the presence of sunlight but dietary sources are important, especially in winter. The disease is characterised by soft bones that bend out of shape and cause deformities. Bones are hardened by the deposition of calcium salts, and this can occur only in the presence of vitamin D. In the UK, many foods, e.g. margarine, are enriched with vitamin D and rickets is relatively uncommon. It may arise where there is a restricted diet or poor nutrition and is treated by giving vitamin D supplements, usually in the form of calciferol.

Ritter's disease a rare infection of the skin caused by staphylococcus bacteria and affecting newborn babies. There is a rash of red spots that begins around the mouth and gradually spreads to other areas. Crusts form and the skin may peel off in layers. The infection must be promptly treated with antibiotics to prevent a fatal outcome.

ROP *see* RETINOPATHY IN PREMATURE BABIES.

roseola infantum, pseudorubella *or* **exanthem subitum** an acute FEVER and skin rash that is highly contagious and affects babies and young children, especially those between the ages of six months and three years. The child suddenly develops a high FEVER of 39.5°–40.5°, for which there is no obvious cause. This usually lasts for three to five days and CONVULSIONS may occur. The child is irritable and generally unwell. The fever normally reaches a peak and then subsides, and this coincides in some, but not all cases, with the development of a red rash, mainly on the chest and abdomen. This normally subsides quite soon and the child feels better. Treatment consists of measures to reduce fever and encouraging the child to drink plenty of fluids. Rarely, e.g. if there have been convulsions accompanying the high temperature or the child has become dehydrated, admittance to hospital may be required. The most common cause is believed to be human herpes virus type 6, although other viruses may be responsible.

rubella *see* GERMAN MEASLES.

rubeola *see* MEASLES.

S

Sabin vaccine, Salk vaccine *see* POLIOVIRUS VACCINE.

St Vitus' dance *see* SYDENHAM'S CHOREA.

sarcoma botryoides a malignant tumour that may arise in young children, occurring in the cervix or vagina of a girl or in the neck of the bladder. Surgery, chemotherapy and radiotherapy may be needed.

scalds *see* BURNS AND SCALDS.

scarlet fever *or* **scarlatina** an infectious disease, now rare in Britain, usually affecting children and characterised by a bright red skin rash. This generally follows a throat infection caused by Streptococcus bacteria, and scarlet fever most commonly arises in children aged two to ten years. Symptoms appear after an incubation period of about three days. There is a high FEVER (up to 104°F or 40°C), chills, headache, VOMITING, rapid pulse and a severe sore throat. The tonsils and lymph glands in the neck are usually swollen and tender. Within 24 hours, a bright red rash appears on the face and spreads to include other parts of the body. The rash fades and disappears after about one week, with peeling of the skin. When it is at its height, the tongue is usually a bright strawberry red, as is the face apart from a pale white area around the mouth. Also characteristic are dark red lines in skin folds and creases. Usually, prompt antibiotic treatment prevents the development of scarlet fever, which was formerly a major cause of death among young children. Both the sore throat and scarlet fever are treated with a course of antibiotics, usually penicillin or erythromycin. The child needs bed rest and must be encouraged to drink plenty of fluids, and full recovery normally occurs within two weeks. Without treatment, serious complications can arise, particularly inflammation of the kidneys (GLOMERULONEPHRITIS), heart (ENDOCARDITIS), middle ear and joints (arthritis or rheumatism).

Scheuermann's disease a disorder of the spine belonging to a group of conditions known as the OSTEOCHONDROSES. It usually becomes apparent during adolescence and is more common in boys than in girls. Symptoms include low back pain and a round-shouldered appearance, with abnormal bending of the thoracic spine (called KYPHOSIS). x-rays reveal the presence of abnormal wedge-shaped vertebral bodies, which are responsible for the deformity of the spine. The cause is unknown but infection, accidental injury, poor circulation during phases of rapid growth or other factors may be implicated. Treatment depends on severity and whether the condition appears to be static or progressive. It may involve physiotherapy, rest and avoidance of activities liable to place stress on the back, orthopaedic and, rarely, surgical treatments.

Schilder's disease a number of severe and progressive neurological disorders that cause increasing physical and intellectual deterioration. They result from the loss of the myelin sheath surrounding nerve tissue in the brain and produce similar effects to those of multiple sclerosis.

schizophrenia in childhood, childhood schizophrenia a mental disorder of childhood that does not appear before the age of seven years and is essentially similar to schizophrenia in teenagers and adults. It is characterised by alterations in behaviour including withdrawal into an autistic-like state, breakdown in thought processes, delusions and hallucinations. It is believed to be brought about by external environmental stresses acting on a child with a predisposition (possibly involving biochemical factors within the brain) towards the condition.

Psychiatric treatment, which may involve hospitalisation, is needed, and certain drugs may be used to control severe symptoms. Ongoing treatment may be needed and the outcome is difficult to predict.

Schönlein-Henoch purpura *or* **Henoch-Schönlein purpura** inflammation of small blood vessels, which is a hypersensitive, allergic reaction and usually occurs in children. It produces skin lesions and rashes on the lower trunk, back and legs, often with pain in the knees and ankles or other joints. There may be blood in urine and stools, but the condition usually resolves itself with time.

school phobia a fear of going to school, degrees of which are relatively common in young children. In its most severe form it is a type of separation anxiety in which the child becomes extremely fearful if parted from the parents. An affected child is usually timid and unsure of himself or herself, lacking self-confidence, emotionally immature and over-dependent on the parents. Such a child may require professional help in order to overcome his or her fears. In less severely affected children, this is normally a transient phase that resolves itself in time with patience and reassurance on the part of the parents and the school.

sclerema neonatorum a usually fatal condition most commonly affecting very ill, premature newborn infants who have become chilled. There is a hardening of the skin and its underlying tissues, which occurs progressively.

scoliosis an abnormal, lateral curving of the spine (from side to side) which can arise as a result of a number of different causes. A slight curvature is common and usually corrects itself naturally as a child grows. However, 1 in 10 children with scoliosis require treatment and in these cases, a prompt diagnosis of the condition is very important. This is because without treatment, the ribcage (and pelvis) can become misaligned and the normal operation of the heart and lungs can then be affected. In 80 per cent of children, the cause of the scoliosis is unknown and in the remaining 20 per cent, it may be due to a congenital disorder of spinal development or a neuromuscular disease. Signs of scoliosis include one shoulder higher than the other, a more prominent hip on one side and difficulty in finding correctly-fitting clothes.

Treatment includes monitoring, with regular x-rays being required to see how the spine is developing. Wearing a back brace may be needed (if the curve exceeds 25 degrees) and this is tailor-made for each child. There may be a requirement for surgery (especially if the curve is greater than 50 degrees) and some children need to wear a plaster jacket or back brace for up to six months after the operation in order to support the spine. Full recovery following surgery can be up to one year.

scrotal defects a baby boy may be born with various CONGENITAL defects of the scrotum, which is the sac or pouch containing the TESTICLES. One or both parts of the scrotum may fail to develop normally, especially in the case of CRYPTORCHIDISM. The former condition is called hemiscrotum. A benign congenital tumour, called a hemangioma, may occur or a hydrocoele (a collection of fluid), and both these conditions may require corrective surgery. Rarely, the penis and the scrotum may be transposed but this can be corrected by surgery.

seatworms *see* THREADWORMS.

secondary sexual characteristics the physical changes appropriate to each sex that develop at PUBERTY.

sedatives *see* DRUG ABUSE.

seizures *see* CONVULSIONS.

separation anxiety signs of anxiety and distress commonly shown by a baby or young child when separated from his or her parents or usual environment or approached by an unfamiliar person.

septal defect of the heart a generally CONGENITAL abnormality of the heart of a newborn baby, affecting the wall or septum that divides either the upper (the atria) or lower (ventricles) chambers. *(See* ATRIAL SEPTAL DEFECT and VENTRICULAR SEPTAL DEFECT.)

severe chronic neutropenia (SCN) a very rare disorder of the blood in which there is a deficiency of white blood cells called neutrophils that form a vital component of the immune system. There are four types of SCN: congenital, idiopathic, autoimmune and cyclical. The congenital form is usually diagnosed soon after birth and an infant is highly susceptible to infections.

In normal health, immature, precursor neutrophils are produced in the bone marrow but in congenital SCN, for some reason they fail to mature. Children with this condition are at high risk of developing LEUKAEMIA. The idiopathic form is of unknown cause and arises in a child who has usually had a normal white blood cell count in the past. It may resolve spontaneously. Autoimmune SCN occurs when the body's immune system attacks its own neutrophils. It is most likely to arise in infancy or early childhood and in most cases, resolves itself over a period of about 1 to 2 years. Cyclical SCN shows a pattern in which the neutrophils go from being almost absent in the blood to reaching a near normal level some 3 weeks later and this reflects a fluctuating rate of production in the bone marrow. with this form of the disorder, the child is most susceptible to infections when the neutrophil count is low.

Diagnosis of the disorder is by means of blood and bone marrow teats and treatment comprises injections of hormone-like chemicals called granulocyte-colony stimulating factors or G-CSFs. Children with the congenital form of the disease are given yearly checks on their bone marrow to look for early signs of leukaemia.

severe combined immunodeficiency (SCID) a group of rare, congenital, inherited disorders affecting white blood cells and the immune system. Three different types of white blood cell can be involved but in all cases, affected children have low immunity and are highly vulnerable to infections and illnesses. SCID can be caused by a defect in one of a number of genes, each of which codes for a particular protein that is vital for the normal development of the immune system. Hence the condition if further classified according to the particular gene that is involved. Also, SCID may be inherited in different ways, either sex-linked and passed on the X-chromosome (a form that only affects boys) or autosomal recessive, affecting both boys and girls but particularly likely to occur when the parents of an affected child are themselves related. This is because the defective gene may be present among members of an extended family without it being apparent, as it is not expressed as an illness because each person also has a healthy copy of the gene as well. But it may then come to light if the abnormal copy of the gene is passed from each carrier parent to their child, enabling the disorder to be expressed. SCID babies may be healthy at birth but infections commonly begin to occur within the first few weeks of life. The infant often feeds poorly and fails to thrive and he or she may have skin rashes and diarrhoea. Usually, a baby is admitted to hospital suffering from a serious infection and SCID is diagnosed during investigations into the cause of the illness. Stringent hygiene precautions and avoidance of infection form a cornerstone of treatment that must be carried out at centres specialising in this disorder.

sex education informing children about all aspects of human reproductive and sexual behaviour in lessons given at school. Formerly in Britain, the reproductive 'facts of life' were taught in biology lessons to all children at about the age of 12 or 13, and this was generally accepted and caused little comment. However, over recent years, the social changes and relaxation of attitudes towards sexual behaviour has meant that sex education has become broader and considerably more controversial. Aspects that cause controversy include the age at which lessons should be started and the moral framework that should support the teaching. Britain has one of the highest rates of teenage pregnancy in the Western world, and some experts believe that the way to reduce this is to introduce sex education at a young age, before children become sexually aware. Some also hold the view that contraceptives should be made freely available to children in order to prevent accidental pregnancies and to limit the spread of sexually transmitted diseases such as HIV. However, others feel that sex education should be given in the context of a strong religious and moral framework, concentrating on the importance of committed relationships, marriage and family. They fear that some children may be encouraged to experiment with sex and may be harmed emotionally, and possibly physically in the process.

Also, in the liberal and permissive sexual climate of today, some young people may be pressured into having sex before they are ready to do so. Another matter that causes controversy is education about homosexuality, particularly whether this should be taught as normal sexual behaviour, reflecting the ambivalent attitude still prevalent towards this aspect of life. Many schools try to steer a middle course through some of the difficulties surrounding sex education by informing and involving parents as much as possible.

sexual abuse of children mistreatment of a child for the purpose of sexual gratification, often perpetrated by an adult but sometimes by an older child upon a younger one. Coercion and intimidation are frequently involved, but also *any* inappropriate fondling of a child amounts to sexual abuse and assault. In recent years, people in many countries including Britain have been forced to acknowledge that sexual abuse of children is a common problem. It often occurs within a family or is carried out by a close friend, relative or other trusted person, and a child may be abused for years before anyone suspects that there may be a problem. Sometimes the abuse comes to light only in adult life, and victims tend to be severely affected, especially when they try to form close relationships of their own. They may have to undergo emotionally painful sessions of therapy to overcome the problems caused by the sexual abuse.

Stringent efforts continue to be made to address the problem and to protect children. Some of the most valuable are in attempting to educate children to report anything wrong that is happening to them, and organisations such as Childline, the NSPCC and Barnardos are invaluable in this respect. All adults in a community, and not just those directly involved in child care, should feel a sense of responsibility for the children in their midst. Anyone who has suspicions that a child is being mistreated or neglected in any way should always report these to an appropriate authority.

SGA *see* GESTATIONAL AGE.

short gut syndrome a CONGENITAL abnormality in which the intestine of a newborn baby is insufficiently developed or too short. The baby fails to thrive because it cannot digest its food properly and hence must be supplied with nutrients by other means (e.g. intravenously). Surgery may be needed or the condition of the intestine may improve with time.

sickle cell anaemia a type of inherited haemolytic anaemia that is genetically determined and that affects people of African ancestry. It is caused by a recessive gene, so people can be carriers of the sickle cell trait without themselves showing any signs of illness. The anaemia occurs in a child who inherits the gene from both parents. The red blood cells have a characteristic, distorted sickle shape, and there are periods of crisis when the anaemia is especially severe. The condition affects babies of both sexes, and symptoms usually become apparent by the age of about six months, the illness then being present for life. The child fails to thrive, has frequent infections and is anaemic, with symptoms of pallor, fatigue, breathlessness and JAUNDICE. There are episodes of joint and bone pain and FEVER, with pains in the hands and feet being especially common. Growth is retarded, and there may be chest and abdominal pains and VOMITING. Skin ulcers may occur, particularly on the ankles, and there are nerve disorders and impairment of the function of the lungs, heart and kidneys. The bones may be distorted and the spleen and heart enlarged.

Treatment is aimed at the relief of symptoms as there is, as yet, no known cure. Blood transfusions may be necessary for severe bouts of anaemia, and drugs used include painkillers and a course of antibiotics to treat infections. Any infection should be treated promptly and immunisations given whenever possible and appropriate. Improved supportive and antibiotic treatment has improved the outlook for sufferers of sickle cell anaemia, but the disease shortens life expectancy, and in adulthood there is a greater risk of stroke and other serious complications. Many people are asymptomatic carriers of the defective gene, which persists at a high level because it confers increased resistance to malaria. Those with a family history of sickle cell anaemia are advised to seek genetic counselling.

SIDS (sudden infant death syndrome) *see* COT DEATH.

sleep terrors sudden awakening from sleep, generally with a cry and extreme fear, confusion and agitation. The child has no recollection of the event once fully awakened. Many children may go through a phase of experiencing sleep terrors but usually this resolves with time.

sleepwalking *or* **somnambulism** leaving the bed and walking about during sleep, sometimes going into another room. The child may respond when spoken to and guided back to bed, but if fully awakened does not remember the events. Many children may go through a phase of sleepwalking but usually this becomes less frequent and then stops altogether with increasing age.

slipped femoral capital epiphysis a condition, most commonly affecting overweight teenage boys, in which the epiphysis of the femur slips out of place at the hip. The condition usually arises slowly and causes pain in the hip which is sometime referred to the knee and thigh. The leg may eventually rotate slightly, and orthopaedic surgery is needed to correct the condition. It is believed to be caused by changes in hormone levels during adolescence. Loss of weight is usually advisable.

smacking *see* DISCIPLINE.

Smith-Magenis syndrome (SMS) a rare, congenital, chromosomal disorder affecting about 1 in every 25,000 newborn babies and characterised by a particular facial appearance, learning difficulties and behavioural problems. It is caused by a micro-deletion of part of chromosome 17, along with its corresponding genes and produces distinctive facial features. There is a broad, flat head with a pronounced forehead, eyes that slant upwards, bushy eyebrows, a flattened nose, puffy lips and a wide mouth. Children often have a hoarse voice and are usually of short stature. Eye disorders such as a squint, partial deafness, SCOLIOSIS, EPILEPSY and heart problems may be present. Peripheral nerve damage causing a lack of sensitivity to pain or heat and cold in the toes and fingers are common features along with an odd gait or muscle weakness. Behavioural difficulties, HYPERACTIVITY and disrupted patterns of sleep are other recognised features. Children also have moderate to severe learning difficulties, with delays in the development of language and other skills. In infancy, it is common for recurrent ear infections to arise and feeding difficulties with poor weight gain may be experienced. Treatment is aimed at relief of the specific physical disorders that accompany the condition along with specialist therapies such as speech therapy and educational/learning support.

smoking children are adversely affected by cigarette smoking in two ways. Firstly, younger children and even the unborn are damaged by parental smoking. A mother who smokes during pregnancy is more likely to have a low birth weight baby or the FOETUS may be damaged during development. Following birth, a smoker's baby is more likely to be a victim of COT DEATH and, in childhood, suffers from more respiratory infections, GLUE EAR and ASTHMA. These children are the victims of the passive smoking of other people's cigarettes. Secondly, children are harmed if they adopt the habit of smoking themselves, which many do at around the age of 11 or 12 onwards. In spite of sustained campaigns warning about the dangers of smoking, many young people are still attracted to the habit, perhaps partly because it is discouraged but also they believe that it makes them seem more grown up. This is in spite of the fact that they usually have to work hard to acquire the habit in the first place, which often causes coughing, nausea, sickness, headaches, etc, when first tried. Health scares appear to have little impact on the young, who have the invincibility of youth; adverse consequences seem to be a lifetime away and too remote to worry about.

Unfortunately, however, many young smokers become addicted and hence become vulnerable to a range of smoking-related illnesses in middle and older age. These include lung CANCER, emphysema, chronic BRONCHITIS, heart attack, stroke and other circulatory disorders. In addition, smoking is a major contributory factor in the development of many other cancers. Tobacco smoke contains 16 known carcinogens (substances capable of causing cancer). Because of its effects on blood circulation, some smokers eventually develop gangrenous limbs, for which the only treatment is amputation. Most develop a COUGH and wheezy breathing and are soon left gasping for breath when they attempt hard physical exertion. In addition, the senses of smell and taste can be considerably reduced and the appearance of the skin and teeth may alter.

solvent abuse *see* DRUG ABUSE.

somatotrophin *see* GROWTH HORMONE.

somnambulism *see* SLEEPWALKING.

'speed' *see* DRUG ABUSE.

spina bifida one of the most common neural tube defects, being a CONGENITAL malformation in a newborn baby in which part of the spinal cord is exposed through a gap in the backbone. Many babies also suffer from HYDROCEPHALUS. A severely affected baby may not survive, and the symptoms usually include paralysis, incontinence, a high risk of MENINGITIS and mental retardation.

Spina bifida usually produces a high level of ALPHA FETOPROTEIN in the amniotic fluid, which can be detected in maternal blood and confirmed by AMNIOCENTESIS.

spinal muscular atrophy (SMA) a genetic disorder of nerve cells causing wastage (atrophy) of the voluntary muscles that direct movements such as walking, head and neck control and swallowing. SMA exists in several different forms with type 1 classed as severe and also known as Werdnig-Hoffmann syndrome. Type 11 is of moderate severity while type 111 is mild, also know as Kugelberg-Werlander disease and only affects children. These three types are all inherited as autosomal, recessive disorders with type 1 generally being apparent at or soon after birth. An affected baby has feeding and breathing difficulties, fails to thrive and usually dies before the age of 2 years. In type 11, symptoms arise in early childhood and there can be considerable physical disabilities as the child grows. In type 111, symptoms may not occur until the teenage years but produce similar disabilities as in type 11. Affected children may require treatment and breathing support along with physiotherapy for musculoskeletal problems.

Sprengel's deformity a CONGENITAL defect of the shoulder blade (scapula), which fails to develop properly. It is abnormally small and displaced and requires corrective surgery.

squinting *see* STRABISMUS.

stammering *or* **stuttering** faltering of normal speech with a repetition of the initial consonant of words. It usually appears in childhood, and nervousness makes the problem worse. However, most children make excellent progress with speech therapy and with sympathetic support and encouragement from family and friends.

Stevens-Johnson syndrome a common hypersensitive reaction to sulphonamide antibiotics that may occur in children, that produces skin lesions, and the eyes and mucosa may ulcerate.

stillbirth the birth of any child who provides no evidence of life.

Still's disease *see* JUVENILE RHEUMATOID ARTHRITIS.

strabismus *or* **squinting** (popularly called crossed eyes) a misalignment of the two eyes, which can be an inherited condition arising in childhood. Various methods are used in treatment, depending on the nature and severity of the condition.

stress it has only recently been recognised that children, like adults, can suffer considerably from the effects of stress. The causes of stress are numerous and include family breakdown, teasing or bullying at school, racial or other abuse and examination pressures. Children may react to stress by showing behavioural changes, such as becoming irritable or withdrawn and moody, or standards of school work may decline. They may not find it easy to talk about what is troubling them, and in extreme cases, a child may become depressed and attempt suicide. It is essential for parents and teachers to be aware of the effects of stress and to help a child to deal with his or her problems. If necessary, professional help should be sought, with the first contact being the family doctor.

stuttering *see* STAMMERING.

sub-acute sclerosing panencephalitis (SSPE) a very rare disease of the brain which is caused by an extreme reaction to the virus that causes MEASLES. It usually arises many years after the original measles infection and causes progressive mental and physical deterioration. It is diagnosed by means of an EEG (electroencephalogram) and by examination of a sample of cerebrospinal fluid obtained via a lumbar puncture. The rate of deterioration can be rapid, occurring over a period of months or much slower, over 10 to 15 years. In both cases, it proceeds inexorably with the child becoming increasingly helpless and unaware and death usually takes place before adulthood is reached. An affected child and his or her family require a great deal of specialist help and support in order to enhance and maintain quality of life for as long as possible.

sucking blisters small, rounded pads that occur on the lips of a young baby and seem to aid sucking. They may be present in a newborn baby if the infant has sucked his or her own thumb or fingers before birth.

sucking pad *see* BUCCAL FAT PAD.

sudden infant death syndrome (SIDS) *see* COT DEATH.

suffocation cessation of breathing, usually caused by some external factor such as smothering, being confined in an airtight space, strangulation, DROWNING, etc. Babies and small children can be at particular risk from various environmental hazards. Well-known examples include plastic bags, which may be pulled over the head, cot pillows, discarded fridges, and any collection of water.

sulfatide lipidosis a rare CONGENITAL, inherited disorder of lipid (fat) metabolism caused by an enzyme deficiency. It causes very severe effects of paralysis and dementia because of a build-up of certain lipids in the central nervous system and other organs. It is usually fatal within about ten years.

sunburn young children have delicate skin and must be protected from the sun. They should be dressed in cool cotton clothing that covers exposed skin and should wear a hat with a brim. Protective sunscreen creams especially formulated for children should also be used. Not only is sunburn extremely painful but there has also been increasing concern in recent years at the rise in the number of cases of skin CANCER in young adults. This is connected with sunburn and exposure to the sun, and it is believed that increasing amounts of UV (ultraviolet) radiation entering the earth's atmosphere through holes in the ozone layer may be responsible. It is believed that even one episode of sunburn in childhood may increase the risk of contracting skin cancer in adult life. Health experts recommend that young children should be kept out of the summer sun between the hours of 11 a.m. and 3 p.m. This is difficult to achieve, especially as children grow older, but parents should at least insist that adequate clothing is worn and sun creams are applied.

supplementary feeding *see* COMPLEMENTARY FEEDING.

supraglottitis *see* ACUTE EPIGLOTTITIS.

Sydenham's chorea *or* **St Vitus' dance** a childhood disorder of the nervous system that is characterised by involuntary, jerky, purposeless movements and is associated with acute rheumatism. The disorder is self-limiting, and symptoms disappear with time, leaving no residual ill-effects. However, about one third of affected children develop chronic rheumatism, which usually involves the heart. The disorder is more likely to occur in children aged over five years, especially girls. Any muscles can be involved but especially those of the face, shoulders and hips. The child contorts the face, and intentional movements are poorly coordinated. The symptoms tend to start slightly and gradually increase, and usually last for between three and eight months. Sometimes the flailing movements of the limbs are so excessive that the child needs to be sedated, but they do not occur during sleep. The symptoms of chorea may appear about six months after a rheumatic infection, particularly RHEUMATIC FEVER.

Treatment consists of rest and possibly mild sedation if movements are especially violent. Reassurance for the child, family and school is vital, and normal life should continue as much as possible. If rheumatism develops or the heart becomes affected, treatment is generally as for rheumatic fever. The cause is thought to be the same streptococcal bacteria responsible for rheumatic disorders but causing an autoimmune response involving the central nervous system. In temperate countries it is more common in the summer and early autumn months, which correlates with the peak incidence of rheumatic fever (in the spring and early summer).

T

talipes *see* CLUBFOOT.

teething the eruption of the 20 first, milk or DECIDUOUS TEETH through the gums in infancy. Teething generally starts around the age of six months, with the incisors at the front of the mouth. The process ends with the appearance of the molars between the ages of 20 to 30 months. Teething commonly causes some distress, which the baby attempts to relieve by biting and rubbing the gums on various objects. There may be fretfulness, excess production of saliva, a flushed appearance and slight FEVER, disturbance of sleep and refusal of meals. These are minor problems that can be relieved with mild analgesics, teething gels and by giving the baby something hard to bite on. It is, however, vital that symptoms of illness in a baby should not be put down to teething when there may be some more serious cause. An ill and feverish child should always be examined by the family doctor.

temper tantrums outbursts of anger, screaming, breath-holding and thrashing about, which are extremely common in toddlers, especially around the age of two. They often result from a child's frustration at not being able to have his or her own way or at being misunderstood at a time when the toddler is trying to assert some degree of independence. Tantrums can be very alarming and annoying for parents, but it is best to remain calm and within reach and ignore the outburst as far as possible. Physical restraint or becoming angry and smacking the child are best avoided (*see* DISCIPLINE). Once the anger subsides, the child may be frightened by his or her outburst and above all needs reassurance and love, but without the parent giving in to the original demand. Tantrums are almost always a passing phase and become less frequent as the child grows older, more capable and open to reason.

testicular cancer a malignant tumour in a testicle of which there are two types, seminoma (arising from the seminiferous epithelium) and teratoma. A teratoma is a tumour composed of unusual tissues not normally found at that site and is derived from partially developed embryological cells. It may develop in a testicle, particularly in one that was undescended, and can occur in boys as young as 15, although it is more common in the 20 to 35 years age group. In recent years there has been an increase in the number of baby boys born with an undescended testicle (CRYPTORCHIDISM), and this condition, even when corrected by early surgery, produces a five-fold greater risk of testicular cancer later on.

Testicular cancer can produce symptoms of an abnormal lump, a dull ache in the groin or abdomen, a feeling of heaviness or more pronounced pain. However, there may also be few or no symptoms. If detected early, the chances of a complete cure are excellent (90 per cent), but treatment may involve surgical removal of the lump or testicle, chemotherapy and/or radiotherapy. It is vital that teenage boys are taught the importance of testicular self-examination, which should be carried out, from the age of 15 years, about once each month. The aim is to become familiar with the normal size, shape and 'feel' of the testicles so that any change is more likely to be noticed. If any irregularity, pain or lump is noticed, the boy must understand the importance of putting aside any feelings of embarrassment, not easy at this age, and see the family doctor. Referral to a specialist is likely to be needed, and most lumps or irregularities are benign.

tetanus *or* **lockjaw** a very serious and potentially fatal infection caused by common soil bacteria called *Clostridium tetani*, which gain access via wounds. All children in the UK are protected by routine immunisation, and tetanus is fortunately now rare. In adult life, booster vaccination against tetanus is needed every ten years.

tetralogy of Fallot a serious CONGENITAL abnormality involving the right side of the heart. It results in unoxygenated blood from the right ventricle entering the aorta, producing symptoms of CYANOSIS and failure to feed and thrive. It is usually detected soon after birth if severe, but may not be diagnosed immediately if less pronounced. Some drugs are usually given to relieve immediate symptoms until surgical repair can be carried out.

threadworms, pinworms *or* **seatworms** (*also called* **enterobiasis** *or* **oxyuriasis**) a common intestinal infestation by parasitic nematode worms, usually occurring in young children. There may be no symptoms, but when they do occur the commonest indication is itching around the anus, especially at night. The child may scratch extensively and cause the skin to become irritated and inflamed. In young girls, the worms may enter the vulva, causing irritation and a discharge. Occasionally, the child may experience abdominal pains and a loss of weight. Rarely, it is possible for the worms to be responsible for an appendicitis. The tiny, nematode worms are only a few millimetres long, and females migrate to the rectum and lay their eggs in the skin around the anus. If the child scratches, the eggs are transferred to the fingers and deposited on toys, clothing, bedding, the toilet seat, etc. The minute microscopic eggs are easily picked up and ingested by another child and remain viable for about three weeks in the environment. They may even be swallowed from the air. The eggs hatch and mature into adult worms in the large intestine and reproduce to begin a new cycle of infestation.

It is extremely rare for them to cause harm, and it is probable that many people have the infestation without realising that this is the case. Symptoms are only likely to occur in young children, and the worms are easily killed by simple drug treatment. All members of the family must receive treatment at the same time, but since reinfestation is common a follow-up dose may be needed. Even without treatment, it is thought that the body rids itself of the worms in time or they die out for reasons that are not known. Maintaining a high standard of hygiene by making sure that children wash their hands and nails, and are discouraged from putting fingers or objects into their mouth, is advisable.

tic a motor tic is an involuntary, short-lived, repetitive movement that does not fulfil any useful function. A phonic or vocal tic is a burst of repetitive, involuntary sound that may or may not include words or phrases. A simple tic involves only a single muscle or one particular sound. A complex tic involves several muscles or a series of sounds. Examples of simple motor tics include rapid blinking, grimacing, nodding and shrugging the shoulders. Complex motor tics include spinning around and reaching out to touch objects or people. Examples of simple phonic tics include grunts and squeaks while complex ones may involve repeating a phrase or making a series of animal sounds. Tics can appear spontaneously, persist for a time and then either disappear again or be replaced by a different tic. There is a great deal of variation in frequency and severity and they are quite common in children aged between 5 and 9 years. Children with certain disorders, especially TOURETTE SYNDROME are particularly likely to exhibit tics. They are usually not damaging but they can appear alarming and embarrassing and a child may become the subject of ridicule or bullying. Hence there is a need for information and understanding of tics among those who have dealings with the child, including his or her school friends. In many children, tics lessen in severity and frequency with age and they may not persist into adult life.

tonsillitis inflammation and infection of the tonsils caused by bacterial or, less commonly, viral infection. The tonsils usually refers to two small masses of lymphoid tissue situated on either side at the back of the mouth in the throat (the palatine tonsils). Another pair, the lingual tonsils, are situated below the tongue while the adenoids are the pharyngeal tonsils, located at the back of the nose. All are part of the body's protective mechanism against infection and are larger in children than in adults. Tonsillitis most commonly affects children after infancy and before PUBERTY.

Symptoms include a severe sore throat that makes swallowing very painful, FEVER and earache. The tonsils are usually swollen and white, as a result of infected material exuding from them, and lymph glands in the neck are enlarged. There is malaise and loss of appetite and, rarely, the development of an abscess on a tonsil. Immediate medical treatment is needed by means of antibiotics, generally penicillin or erythromycin, along with pain relief. Complete bed rest is advisable and the child should be encouraged to drink plenty of fluids. Considerable coaxing may be needed as swallowing is very painful. Iced drinks and sipping with a straw may be helpful. Recovery is usually good and complete within about one week or ten days. In some cases a child may suffer recurrent bouts of tonsillitis and the tonsils and adenoids may become permanently enlarged so that breathing is affected. If this occurs, surgery to remove the tonsils (tonsillectomy) and adenoids (adenectomy) may become necessary. In the case of abscess on a tonsil, admittance to hospital for surgery may well be necessary.

TOPV (trivalent live oral polio vaccine) *see* POLIOVIRUS VACCINE.

torsion of a testicle twisting or rotation of the spermatic cord and testicle, leading to irreversible damage if not treated promptly. It is most common in boys and young men between the ages of 12 and 20 and usually affects only one side. The symptoms may arise for no apparent cause or as a result of strenuous physical activity. They include severe pain in the testicle with swelling, reddening and hardening of the scrotum, nausea, VOMITING, FEVER, sweating and rapid heartbeat. This is a medical emergency requiring immediate treatment in hospital. Treatment is by means of corrective surgery to attach the testicle to the wall of the scrotum to prevent a recurrence. The unaffected testicle may be similarly fixed at the same time as a precaution. Recovery is normally excellent.

The cause may not be apparent and torsion is sometimes present at birth. If treatment is delayed, the blood supply to the testicle may become cut off so that the organ is irreversibly damaged. In this case, surgical removal is needed but the remaining testicle produces sufficient hormones to ensure sexual maturation and fertility.

toxocariasis a disease caused by a parasitic infestation with the larvae of roundworms that commonly infect dogs (*Toxocara canis*) or cats (*Toxocara cati*). The parasites are passed to people, particularly young children, by swallowing eggs that are deposited in the faeces of infected pets. There are a variety of symptoms depending on which tissues are affected and whether allergic reactions take place. They include eye lesions and uveitis (an inflammation of the uveal tract of the eye, the iris, choroid and ciliary body). This usually occurs as the sole symptom when the infestation has been with just a few larvae. There may also be wheezing, COUGH, symptoms of PNEUMONIA and lung inflammation, enlargement of the liver and spleen, blood changes and skin rash. Muscular pains, VOMITING, FEVER and CONVULSIONS may also be present.

If symptoms are confined to the eyes, treatment is by means of corticosteroids alone. Drugs that may be prescribed for other manifestations include mebendazole (vermox), prednisone and diethylcarbamazine. The activity of the parasites and the course of the disease last for about six to 18 months when the larvae die off and do not mature into adult worms. Hence the outlook is generally good, although the lesions produced by the larvae may remain.

Young children are particularly vulnerable through the habit of putting their hands in their mouths and also, possibly, because their immune system is immature. The eggs of the parasite persist for a long time in the environment, long after the faeces have rotted away. Hence any ground frequented by dogs and cats should be regarded as suspect. After the eggs have been swallowed by the child, the larvae hatch in the intestine and pass into the blood circulation. They disperse and lodge in other tissues and organs in the body and may cause considerable damage and allergic reactions. The body responds to the presence of the larvae by producing a form of scar tissue (called granulation tissue). In the eye, this causes the formation of a small nodule or nodules known as granulomas. It is estimated that about 2 per cent of people in the UK may be affected by the parasite but many do not exhibit symptoms. Preventative measures include worming pets regularly and excluding them from play areas and covering children's sand pits, and also by making sure that children always wash their hands, including beneath the nails, after playing outside or handling pets, particularly before eating or drinking.

toxoplasmosis *see* CONGENITAL TOXOPLASMOSIS.

tracheo-oesophageal fistula *see* **oesophageal atresia**.

tranquillisers *see* DRUG ABUSE.

transient tachypnea of the newborn (TTNB) *or* **neonatal wet lung syndrome** a condition resulting from slow resorption of the fluid in the lungs of a newborn baby which is naturally present before birth. Resorption of fluid usually occurs during labour so that when the baby is born it is able to fill and expand the lungs. TTNB is more likely to arise in a baby who has been delivered by emergency CAESARIAN SECTION, and it causes symptoms of rapid breathing movements, grunting, shortage of oxygen in the blood and possibly CYANOSIS. The baby requires special care, nursing and oxygen but normally recovers well within two or three days.

transposition of the great arteries a CONGENITAL abnormality in which the aorta (the main artery of the body) arises directly from the right instead of the left ventricle (lower larger chamber). The pulmonary artery arises abnormally from the left instead of the right ventricle. The newborn baby immediately develops severe CYANOSIS and acidosis because of the breakdown in normal circulation. A technique known as balloon atrial septostomy must be immediately carried out and certain drugs may be given to improve the baby's condition. However, early corrective surgery usually needs to be performed.

travel sickness *see* MOTION SICKNESS.

triplets a multiple birth of three infants following a single pregnancy.

trisomy a group of CONGENITAL conditions in which one extra chromosome is present in each body cell, i.e. 47 instead of the normal 46. The extra chromosome is a duplicate of one of a normal pair and may involve 8, 13, 18, 21 (DOWN'S SYNDROME) or 23 (the sex chromosomes). People born with these conditions usually suffer a range of physical and intellectual disabilities that may be very severe.

trivalent live oral polio vaccine (TOPV) *see* POLIOVIRUS VACCINE.

TTNB *see* TRANSIENT TACHYPNEA OF THE NEWBORN.

Turner's syndrome a CONGENITAL genetic disorder of females in which there is only one X- (sex) chromosome instead of the usual two. Hence those affected have 45 instead of 46 chromosomes, the ovaries are absent and secondary sexual characteristics fail to develop. The child is of short stature and may have webbing of the neck and other developmental defects. The heart may be affected and there can be DEAFNESS and intellectual impairment. In a less severe form, the second X-chromosome is present but is abnormal, lacking some of the usual genetic material.

twin a multiple birth of two infants following a single pregnancy. The babies may be MONOZYGOTIC or DIZYGOTIC twins.

U

umbilical cord the cord connecting a FOETUS to the placenta, containing two arteries and one vein. It is approximately 60 cm long and is severed after birth, when it shrivels to a stump that falls off to leave a mark, the navel or umbilicus. At the present time, there is considerable interest in harvesting stem cells from umbilical cords for transplantation to patients suffering from certain serious medical conditions.

umbilical hernia *or* **omphalocele** a bulging out of a greater or smaller proportion of abdominal digestive organs in the region of the umbilicus. It is a CONGENITAL condition, caused by a weakness in the abdominal wall at the base of the umbilical cord, and the bulge is covered by a thin layer of membrane. The protrusion is covered by sponges soaked in sterile saline, or the baby's lower body may be enclosed in a bag containing this solution. The condition is usually treated with early corrective surgery.

under-age drinking *see* ALCOHOL.

underdeveloped left ventricle syndrome a serious CONGENITAL heart condition that arises in a newborn baby two or three days after birth, as the ductus arteriosus (a blood vessel that operates in the FOETUS) closes over. Most babies with this syndrome do not survive, although new treatment techniques, including transplantation, may prove helpful.

undescended testicle *see* CRYPTORCHIDISM.

unilateral renal agenesis *see* KIDNEY DEFECTS.

ureter, defects of the ureters are a pair of tubes joining each kidney to the bladder. Various CONGENITAL abnormalities may arise in a newborn baby which are usually associated with kidney anomalies. They include an extra or displaced ureter, abnormally placed openings, blockage or stricture and hernia (ureterocele), Many of these conditions require corrective surgery.

urethra, defects of the urethra is the duct that carries urine from the bladder out of the body and passes through the penis in males. Various CONGENITAL abnormalities may arise in a newborn baby, some of which have been described elsewhere (*see* HYPOSPADIAS, EPISPADIAS). Constriction or stenosis may occur, which is treated by surgical correction. Also 'urethral valves' may arise, formed from folds of tissue, particularly in boys, which causes blockages. This also requires prompt corrective surgery to prevent damage and infection.

urticaria *or* **nettle rash** an allergic hypersensitive reaction to some environmental substance, food or drug, causing a rash and intensely itchy skin. It can occur at any age but may be extremely distressing for children. The child may require antihistamine preparations prescribed by the family doctor, and the causal substance, if this is known, should be avoided.

Usher syndrome (USH) a rare, inherited, genetic disorder that causes deterioration in hearing and vision which may progress to total deafness and blindness and affects 1 in every 25,000 children. Several genes are involved and at least three types of the syndrome are recognised. In type 1 (USH 1), a baby is born deaf and his or her sense of balance is involved so that normal development and acquirement of skills such as sitting up, crawling and walking are often delayed. Deterioration in vision usually starts by the age of 10 years and it may progress rapidly to complete blindness in a short space of time. In type 2 (USH 2), the baby is usually born with moderate to severe hearing loss but is not totally deaf. Hearing aids can be useful and the sense of balance is unaffected. Deterioration in vision may not begin until adult life in this form of the condition. In type 3 (USH3), the baby is born with normal vision and hearing and there is no deterioration in either of these senses during childhood. Early diagnosis and intervention helps to preserve hearing and vision for as long as possible and aids the child's development and ability to learn. However, there is currently no cure for USH. There are many helpful, sophisticated devices (such as cochlear implants) that can prove helpful in enabling the child to deal with the disabilities produced by the disorder.

V

valvular heart disease any disease or condition affecting the valves of the heart, particularly the aortic and mitral valves. Children may have CONGENITAL valve disease or it may arise as a result of infection, particularly rheumatic illnesses. These conditions are usually treated with drugs and surgery, depending on the nature and severity of the disease.

varicella *see* CHICKEN POX.

vasculitis vasculitis simply means inflammation of blood vessels. There are numerous different kinds, depending upon the size of the blood vessels that are involved and their location and distribution within the body. A variety of illnesses and disorders can produce vasculitis and depending upon type, a range of symptoms may be present. These include disturbance of vision (if blood vessels in the retina are involved), red spots visible in the skin which may be small (petuchiae) or larger (purpura), headaches (either due to inflammation of blood vessels in the brain or caused by vision disturbance), aching and/or swelling and pain in joints, kidney problems and high blood pressure, abdominal pains and bloating, heart pain and angina, breathing problems, fever and chest pain. The most common forms of vasculitis in children are KAWASAKI DISEASE and HENOCH-SCONLEIN

PURPURA. These conditions are usually fairly easy to diagnose but rarer forms of childhood vasculitis can be more difficult to pin down. Treatment depends upon severity, type and underlying cause. Severe cases usually require hospital admittance involving powerful drugs that must be given under specialist supervision.

velocardial facial syndrome *or* **Shprintzen syndrome** an inherited, genetic, chromosomal disorder in which there is a deletion of a minute part of chromosome 22 and affecting about 1 in every 2,000 children. It produces a range of symptoms that vary in severity, including learning difficulties, psychiatric problems, behavioural problems, ATTENTION DEFICIT DISORDER, INGUINAL HERNIA, immune system disorders, ear problems, CLEFT PALATE, and heart abnormalities. There is a typical appearance, the features of which include short stature, thin fingers and hands, a small head, an open, small mouth and narrow eyes. The condition cannot be cured and treatment is aimed at the physical manifestations along with appropriate provision of behavioural and learning support.

ventouse *or* **vacuum extraction** a method of assisted delivery of a baby by means of a suction cap attached to the head on which gentle, steady pressure is exerted.

ventricular septal defect (VSD) a CONGENITAL heart defect in a newborn baby in which there are one or more abnormal openings through the septum or membrane that should normally separate the two ventricles (lower chambers of the heart). Depending on severity, it may be diagnosed within the first few weeks of life with the development of degrees of heart failure. It is treated by means of anticongestive measures and strict, prompt treatment of infections in the first instance and then by means of corrective surgery, if necessary.

vernix caseosa a greasy, whitish secretion on the skin of a FOETUS and newborn baby.

version turning a baby in late pregnancy into a position better suited for delivery.

verruca another term for a WART but usually referring to one that occurs on the foot and commonly occurs in children. The causal virus is often contracted from swimming pool changing room floors and the verruca should be treated by applications of solutions prescribed by the family doctor.

vesico-ureteric reflux (VUR) an abnormal condition in which the valves that usually prevent the backflow of urine from the bladder into the ureters (the pair of tubes that lead from each kidney to the bladder) fail to work properly. In severe cases, urine flows backwards as far as the kidneys causing them to swell and become enlarged (HYDRONEPHROSIS). VUR arises in 1 in every 100 children and may be diagnosed at, or shortly after birth or be suspected when a child has repeated urinary tract infections. It is diagnosed and monitored by two scanning techniques ultrasound and voiding cysto-urethrogram (VCUG).

The condition is initially treated by monitoring and courses of antibiotics but some children may require surgery (called ureteric re-implantation). The operation involves severing the ureters from their attachment point and then re-attaching them at an angle to the bladder to recreate 'valves' to prevent the backflow of urine.

volvulus neonatorum a twisting of the bowel causing an obstruction in a newborn baby that produces symptoms of pain, abdominal swelling, non-passage of faeces and VOMITING and must be treated immediately by surgery.

vomiting the reflex action in which the stomach contents are expelled through the mouth because of the contraction of the diaphragm and abdominal wall muscles. It is a very common symptom of a variety of childhood illnesses and infections. Recurrent vomiting can rapidly lead to the development of DEHYDRATION in a small child and should always be reported to the doctor.

Von Recklinghausen's disease (neurofibromatosis) a CONGENITAL disorder in which soft tissue tumours form along nerves and beneath the skin. These tumours can be large and pendulous, and there are often other anomalies such as decalcification of bones, fibrosis of the lungs and formation of kidney stones. One well-known victim was the 'Elephant Man', who lived in England during the 1800s.

VSD *see* VENTRICULAR SEPTAL DEFECT.

W

wart a solid benign growth in the skin caused by a virus. They are infecious and spread rapidly in schools, etc. They often disappear spontaneously but can be dealt with in several ways, e.g. by cryosurgery (freezing), laser treatment and electrocautery. (*See also* VERRUCA.)

Werdrug-Hoffman disease an uncommon inherited disorder in which there is degeneration of cells in the spinal cord and brainstem. Symptoms usually appear in infancy and include floppiness, lack of sucking ability and stretch reflexes, paralysis, fine twitches of the tongue and other muscles and swallowing difficulties.

West's syndrome *or* **infantile spasms** a brain disorder affecting about 1 baby in every 5,000 under 12 months of age. It is characterised by the occurrence of infantile spasms that are a form of EPILEPSY, accompanied by delayed development and often, significant learning disabilities. An EEG (electroencephalogram) that records brain waves shows a characteristic pattern known as hypsarrhythmia. However, it is possible for a child to suffer from infantile spasms without the hypsarrhythmia that is characteristic of West's syndrome. In many cases the disorder is congenital and the cause may be a developmental brain abnormality, a metabolic disease or a genetic/chromosomal disorder (especially tuberous sclerosis). Other causes include severe brain damage at birth. However, in a quarter of all cases, no obvious cause can be found. Spasms usually begin around the age of 6 months and they take a particular form, with a rapid jerk and forward, bowing movement (sometimes described as 'salaam spasms'). They often occur in bouts with just a few seconds between each jerk and they can make the child irritable and unsettled. However, although distressing to watch, the spasms do not cause brain damage and usually, they have ceased by the age of 2 years. Unfortunately, many children go on to develop other types of seizure and often there is learning disability which varies in severity.

Treatment is by means of drugs to lessen the occurrence and severity of the spasms and in a small number of children, brain surgery can be helpful. A range of therapies along with educational/learning support are other methods used to help the child to reach his or her full potential and to enhance quality of life.

whooping cough *or* **pertussis** an infectious disease of childhood, caused by the bacterium *Bordetalla pertussis*, which produces a characteristic COUGH and other respiratory symptoms. As a result of immunisation, the incidence and severity of the illness are generally less than was formerly the case, although children do occasionally develop a whooping-type cough. The mucous membranes lining the air passages are affected, and after a one or two week incubation period, FEVER, catarrh and a cough develop. The cough then becomes paroxysmal, with continual bouts lasting up to one minute. At the end of each bout the child draws in the breath with a characteristic whooping sound. After about two weeks the symptoms begin to subside, although the cough may persist for some time. Subsequent respiratory infections may produce a similar paroxysmal type of cough, although this is not a recurrence of whooping cough itself. Treatment is by means of bed rest, pain relief and plenty of drinks, with the child being kept isolated from others while symptoms are at their height. DEHYDRATION may be a danger if the child is continually sick. In general, antibiotics are not recommended, except for infants who are seriously ill or patients with complications, in which case hospital treatment is usually necessary. Whooping cough can be serious in small children aged less than two years who may develop ASPHYXIA, broncho-pneumonia and CONVULSIONS. Other serious complications include rupture of blood vessels in the brain (cerebral haemorrhage) or eye, retinal detachment caused by the violent coughing, TUBERCULOSIS and ENCEPHALITIS (inflammation of the brain). Some children may sustain lung damage, leading to emphysema or ASTHMA. Such severe complications can result in permanent brain damage or death, and all children (with rare exceptions) should be protected by vaccination.

William's syndrome a rare, congenital, genetic disorder caused by the absence (deletion) of a gene located on chromosome 7. In normal health, this gene codes for a protein that is important in building the structure of the walls of blood vessels, enabling contraction and expansion and conferring strength. The abnormality affects about 1 in every 10,000 to 25,000 newborn babies but it is not thought to be inherited but rather to arise as a spontaneous mutation in the individual concerned. Affected children commonly suffer from heart and circulatory problems (due to abnormal narrowing of blood vessels) as well as musculo-skeletal disorders and kidney problems. They exhibit characteristic facial features which include a small jaw, narrow head, eyes that are widely spaced, a turned-up nose, irregular teeth and a wide mouth. The hearing may be sensitive so that the child is easily startled. Learning difficulties, problems with balance and coordination, incessant chattering, hyperactivity and sleep disorders are other commonly recognised features. Diagnosis is made by means of a blood test and babies are often of low birth weight, poor at feeding and slow to gain weight and reach developmental milestones, including acquisition of language skills. Treatment is aimed at the specific problems that may be present, along with appropriate therapies and learning/educational support.

Wilm's tumour *or* **congenital nephroblastoma** a malignant tumour of the kidney that is present at birth and is usually diagnosed in children aged under five years. Occasionally symptoms may appear later in childhood or, rarely, in adults. The usual presenting symptom is an abdominal mass that can be felt through the skin. There may be FEVER, pain in the abdomen, blood in urine, loss of appetite and weight, VOMITING and nausea. Diagnosis and treatment involve admittance to hospital, with surgical removal of the diseased kidney, chemotherapy and possibly radiotherapy. Younger children have a slightly more favourable prognosis, but this is a severe condition that cannot always be cured.

Wiskott-Aldrich syndrome a recessive disorder carried on the X-chromosome that affects the immune system, causing blood changes, ECZEMA and increased likelihood of infections and certain types of CANCER.

witch's milk a secretion that may occasionally be exuded from the nipples of a newborn baby if levels of maternal lactating hormone have been high before birth.

word blindness a popular term for DYSLEXIA.

X

X-chromosome the sex chromosome present in males and females. Females have two (XX) and males one (XY). Certain disorders such as HAEMOPHILIA are carried on the X-chromosome. Occasionally, one or more extra X-chromosome may be present in a female (triple X syndrome). These often produce degrees of intellectual retardation. (*See* KLINEFELTER'S SYNDROME.)

X-linked agammaglobulinaemia (XLA) *or* **Bruton's sex-linked aggamaglobulinaemia** a rare, inherited, genetic disorder affecting the immune system. It is caused by abnormalities in a gene carried on the X-chromosome that codes for the enzyme Bruton's tyrosine kinase (Btk). There is a failure in the maturation of certain white blood cells and in the production of gammaglobulin, vital for the formation of antibodies to fight off infections. Girls can be carriers of XLA but only boys can have the disorder, which is characterised by the occurrence of severe, recurrent bacterial infections. There may also be enlarged tonsils, adenoids and other lymph glands, along with swelling of joints. Treatment comprises antibiotics to combat infections and regular injections of immunoglobulin (antibody replacement therapy). It is important for the child to avoid the risk of infection whenever possible and for all infections to be promptly treated with antibiotics.

X-linked mental retardation *or* **fragile X syndrome** a genetic defect of the X-chromosome that affects only males. It causes mental retardation and may be linked with AUTISM. Physical manifestations include enlarged ears and testicles along with a prominent chin and forehead. The X-chromosome is fragile and may fragment, and the condition may be quite a common cause of intellectual disability.

Y

Y-chromosome the small sex chromosome that confers maleness. Normal males have 22 matched pairs of chromosomes and one unmatched pair of one X and one Y-chromosome, making 46 in all. Occasionally, the Y-chromosome may be repeated, giving a complement of 47 chromosomes, a condition known as 47 XYY syndrome. This may produce some intellectual and learning disabilities in affected boys.